The Cardio Shift

Transform Your Heart Health with the Revolutionary Intermittent Fasting and Exercise Protocol

BSK Publishing

For more information or to contact us directly:
http://www.vicky-prospect-heathcare.com

ISBN - Paperback: 978-1-998585-16-8

DISCLAIMER

The content provided in this book is designed to provide helpful information on the subjects discussed. This book is not meant to be used, nor should it be used, to diagnose or treat any medical condition. The claims in this book are theoretical and to be used for illustrative purposes only. The publisher and the authors are not responsible for any actions you take or do not take as a result of reading this book, and are not liable for any damages or negative consequences from action or inaction to any person reading or following the information in this book. References are provided for informational purposes only and do not constitute endorsement of any websites or other sources. Readers should also be aware that the websites listed in this book may change or become obsolete.

Acknowledgements

I dedicate this book to my beloved children, who have stood by me as my unwavering pillars of strength throughout my adult life. My first daughter, Joyce, has been a steadfast presence, offering her love and support from her earliest years, and now, as a mature woman, she continues to serve families with compassion and dedication as a social worker. Charles, my second child, fills me with immense pride. At a young age, he ventured abroad for his studies and excelled, earning the marks to become a highly skilled engineer. Vera, my middle child, has always inspired me with her dedication to her education and her remarkable discipline as a teenager. Her perseverance earned her a place in medical school, a reflection of her strong character and determination. Lastly, Faith, my youngest daughter, has been my spirited one, full of energy and potential. Despite challenges, her talents are undeniably inspirational. She is a gifted artist, an excellent mathematician, and a well-rounded individual who inspires those around her with her abilities in art, music, sports, and technology. I remain eternally grateful to each of my children for the hope, strength, and love they have brought into my life.

After completing my BSc Hons degree at St. George's Medical School in London, I began my career as a nurse at the heart attack treatment center at Imperial College London. It was there that my manager, Naomi, recognized my potential and believed that I could achieve more. She provided me with a reference that enabled me to pursue a master's degree in cardiology. That advanced education expanded my knowledge in the field and allowed me to inspire both my colleagues and my family with my newfound expertise.

However, life is often marked by unexpected challenges. In the midst of my career, tragedy struck when I lost my stepfather, the man who had raised me and nurtured my academic aspirations. His passing was a devastating blow, but it also opened my eyes to the significant knowledge gap in the field of cardiology, especially in Cameroon. Returning to bury him, I saw the urgent need for awareness and preventive measures in heart disease, which inspired me to establish the Heart Alert Foundation. Through this initiative, I sought to educate people about the risks of cardiovascular disease and the importance of prevention, focusing on raising awareness of heart conditions and their risk factors.

At the same time, my children were growing fast, and as a single parent, I knew that they needed me. I made the conscious decision to prioritize their upbringing, to be there for them in every important moment, and to support them as they grew into the remarkable individuals they are today.

As I approached my fiftieth year, I began to feel an emotional void, a longing for the connection I had never had with my biological father. I embarked on a search for him, and when I finally found him, I discovered that he had been suffering from type 2 diabetes for many years. This revelation led me to get tested, and I was informed that I was prediabetic, with an HbA1c of 46mmol/L. Unfortunately, at that time, I did not have the depth of knowledge I now possess about preventive medicine, and as time passed, my HbA1c levels rose to 53mmol/L. I could not help but wish that I had found my father sooner so that I could have helped him manage his health, but sadly, he passed away the same year I made contact, before I had the chance to truly know him.

Determined not to let the same fate befall me, I embarked on a personal journey to reverse my diabetes, following the program outlined in this book. Through intermittent fasting, a low-carbohydrate diet, and consistent exercise, I set a goal of losing 10% of my body weight in three months. I am proud to say that I lost 4kg in the first month, and I am committed to continuing this journey toward better health. I invite you to join me on this path, and I encourage you to look out for my second book, which will chronicle my ongoing journey with diabetes.

In addition to my personal health journey, I decided to return to my studies, seeking to deepen my understanding of cardiovascular disease. I enrolled at the University of South Wales via the Learner platform to obtain a master's degree in preventive cardiovascular medicine. With the knowledge and skills I have acquired, I now feel empowered and well-equipped to help others live a life free from the burden of cardiovascular disease.

I firmly advocate for preventive medicine rather than focusing solely on curative measures. Cardiovascular disease, in many cases, is a lifestyle condition, and by adopting lifestyle interventions, we can significantly reduce the risk of heart disease. The suffering that comes with illness, the pain, the limitations, the days lost from work, is not inevitable if we take action to prevent it. The financial costs, both to individuals and to the economy, can be staggering, but they are costs we do not have to bear if we embrace a proactive approach to health.

I extend my deepest thanks to each and every one of you who has taken the time to read this book. By doing so, you are taking an important first step toward claiming your freedom to live a healthier, more fulfilling life, free from the constraints of cardiovascular disease.

Table of Contents

The Silent Killer: Cardiovascular Disease

The prevalence and impact of cardiovascular disease worldwide

Cardiovascular disease remains one of the most formidable health challenges across the globe. Known for its quiet and often unnoticed progression, it has rightfully earned the nickname "the silent killer." The disease affects millions of people, making it a leading cause of death worldwide. It not only shortens lives but also impacts the quality of life significantly. Recognizing its prevalence is the first step in combating its reach. This disease does not discriminate, affecting individuals of all backgrounds and ages, though it is more prevalent in adults over 40. This is why it is crucial for you, especially if you are in this age group or approaching it, to be aware of and actively manage your heart health.

The impact of cardiovascular disease extends beyond the individual. It weighs heavily on families, communities, and even countries' economies due to high medical costs and loss of productivity. The cost of treatments, hospital stays, and medications can be overwhelming, not to mention the personal toll and stress it places on the patients and their loved ones. Therefore, understanding this impact can further motivate one to take preventative or management actions towards their heart health.

Managing heart health is not just about prolonging life; it's about improving the quality of those extra years. The heart, a vital organ, needs care and attention, much like any critical component of a well-functioning system. Understanding heart health involves recognizing the signs of heart problems, knowing the lifestyle factors that can influence heart health, and being aware of the necessary steps to take to mitigate risks. This is particularly important as you age, as the risk of developing heart-related issues increases.

Preventative measures such as regular exercise, maintaining a healthy diet, and monitoring cholesterol and blood pressure can significantly reduce the risk of heart disease. Moreover, for those already diagnosed with cardiovascular conditions, managing these factors becomes not just a preventative measure but a crucial part of everyday life to avoid further complications.

Part of managing your heart health efficiently is becoming informed. Knowledge truly is power when it comes to dealing with cardiovascular disease. By understanding the disease's workings, its triggers, and its effects on your body, you can make informed decisions that lead to a healthier heart. These informed decisions range from choosing the right foods, engaging in appropriate exercise, and even knowing when to seek medical intervention.

The goal of this book is not only to inform but to transform your approach to heart health. It aims to provide you with practical, actionable steps that you can integrate seamlessly into your daily life. The focus is on creating a sustainable and enjoyable lifestyle that supports the health of your heart, enabling you to live your life to the fullest. Remember, taking care of your heart is not just about avoiding disease; it's about creating a robust foundation for an active and joyous life.

As you continue reading, keep in mind that each piece of information is a stepping stone to becoming an advocate for your health. This book will equip you with the necessary tools and knowledge, turning the concern of heart disease into proactive and preventive health management. Embrace this journey with a positive mindset, and let's take the first steps towards a heart-healthy lifestyle together.

A Personal Journey: Confronting Cardiovascular Disease

Heart disease often appears as more than just a personal health issue; it often affects entire families across generations. It becomes a pattern, observed and experienced as relatives face similar health challenges and sometimes premature deaths. Understanding this can trigger a profound sense of urgency and responsibility, to make changes not just for personal health but for the benefit of our entire family line.

It's hard to watch someone you love suffer from health issues, especially when those issues are severe like heart disease. The pain is compounded when it leads to losing them. Witnessing such losses within a family can evoke a strong resolve to prevent the same fate for oneself and one's children. This is a natural response, driven by both love and fear.

The impact of such losses is deep and far-reaching. It extends beyond immediate grief to shape our attitudes towards our own health and lifestyle choices. It raises important questions: How can we avoid the same fate? What can be done differently? This is where the journey often begins for many, in the search for answers and solutions to break this cycle of familial heart disease.

Resolving to break the cycle of heart disease is not merely a decision. It's a commitment to life, to family, and to community. This commitment starts with education and understanding. Knowing what contributes to heart disease and how it can be prevented or managed is fundamental. The next step is translating this knowledge into action, adopting lifestyle changes that promote heart health, advocating for regular health check-ups, and encouraging open discussions about health within the family.

Protecting your community becomes a natural extension of protecting your family. It starts with sharing your journey, the lessons learned, the changes made, and the benefits observed. It involves being a role model and a source of support, encouraging others to take heart health seriously and to take proactive steps towards healthier habits.

This section of the book aims to provide you, the reader, with both the information and the inspiration needed to undertake this transformation. It will guide you through understanding the risks and the strategies to mitigate them. It's about making informed choices and taking definitive actions towards a healthier heart, not just for yourself but also for those around you.

By choosing to confront familial heart disease head-on, you are taking a powerful stand. You are not only increasing your own chances of a longer, healthier life but are also contributing to the health and well-being of your community. This proactive approach can create a ripple effect, encouraging others to also take their heart health seriously. It's a journey of empowerment, for yourself and for your loved ones.

Every step you take on this journey is a step toward a healthier heart and a healthier family. Whether it's choosing to eat healthier, exercising more, managing stress effectively, or quitting smoking, each choice is pivotal. It's these choices that can rewrite your family's heart health history, paving the way for a healthier future for generations to come.

So let this section not only serve as a reflection on the past losses due to heart disease but more importantly, as a proactive blueprint for a heart-healthy lifestyle that breaks the cycle of familial heart disease. It's about turning grief into action and fear into empowerment.

Together, step by step, change can happen. Let's embark on this journey not just with hope but with determination. A heart-healthy life is not just a possibility; with the right knowledge and actions, it becomes a probability.

A Comprehensive Approach to Heart Health

Heart health is essential. Everyone knows it's important to keep the heart healthy, especially as we age. For adults over 40, managing or preventing cardiovascular disease is crucial for longevity and a better quality of life. There are many ways to maintain heart health, but let's focus on a very effective approach: combining intermittent fasting, exercise, and lifestyle changes.

Intermittent fasting is a method of eating that cycles between periods of fasting and eating. It's not about which foods to eat, but rather when you should eat them. This approach has gained popularity due to its simplicity and the significant benefits it can offer for heart health. Research shows that intermittent fasting can improve blood pressure, cholesterol levels, reduce inflammation, reverse pre-diabetes and type two diabetes. These are all risk factors for cardiovascular disease. The idea is that during fasting, the body exhausts its sugar stores and starts burning fat. This process can lead to weight loss and improved metabolic health, a key factor in cardiovascular disease prevention.

Exercise is another cornerstone of cardiovascular health. Regular physical activity helps maintain the fitness of the heart, lungs, and blood vessels. It can also help lower your blood pressure, boost your levels of good cholesterol, reverse your diabetes and improve blood flow. The best part? You don't need to engage in intense workouts. Brisk walking, swimming, or cycling at a moderate pace can be hugely beneficial. The key is consistency. Aim for at least 150 minutes of moderate-intensity aerobic exercise per week. This can be broken down into 30-minute sessions over five days a week.

Lastly, lifestyle changes encompass a wide range of activities and decisions which contribute to the overall quality of your health. This includes getting adequate sleep, managing stress, choosing healthier foods,reducing alcohol and quitting smoking. Each of these factors plays a crucial role in heart health. Sleep, for instance, helps heal and repair your heart, blood vessels and essential organs. An adult should aim for 7-9 hours of quality sleep per night. Stress management is also vital, as excessive stress can lead to heart issues. Techniques like mindfulness, meditation, and deep breathing can reduce stress and enhance your heart's health.

Combining these three elements intermittent fasting, regular exercise, and healthy diet. creates a powerful and effective plan for cardiovascular health. This approach is not just about avoiding disease. It's about creating a robust framework for long-term health and vitality. It requires commitment and a shift in lifestyle, but the benefits are well worth it.

Let's break down how you can start integrating these components into your daily routine. First, consult with a healthcare provider before starting any new diet or exercise program, especially if you have existing health issues. Once you have the green light, start by introducing intermittent fasting gradually. Begin with shorter fasting periods of 16 hours and slowly extend them to 24 hours. For exercise, find activities you enjoy. This makes it easier to stick to a routine. Lastly, assess your current lifestyle and pinpoint areas where you could make healthier choices. Small, incremental changes can lead to substantial improvements over time.

Remember, the goal is to make these practices a regular part of your life. Patience and persistence are key. It might seem challenging at first, but by steadily working on these areas, you'll notice improvements not just in your cardiovascular health, but also in your overall well-being.

The journey to better heart health is a personal one. Each person's body responds differently to dietary changes, types of exercise, and lifestyle adjustments. It is essential to tailor these elements to fit your individual needs and preferences. Tracking your progress can also be incredibly motivating. Keep a log of your fasting hours, physical activity, and lifestyle changes, and note how your body responds. This personalized plan, backed by science, is not just about preventing or managing disease, it's about empowering you to take control of your health and live your life to the fullest.

In conclusion, heart health is not governed by one single activity or habit but by a combination of various factors that include diet, exercise, and overall lifestyle. By understanding and applying the principles of intermittent fasting, engaging in regular physical activity, and making positive lifestyle changes, you are taking significant strides towards not only improving your heart health but enhancing your overall vitality. This comprehensive approach is your pathway to a healthier heart and a fuller, more vibrant life.

Empowering You to Take Control

Heart health is essential. It determines how you live your day-to-day life. Good heart health means more energy, better mood, and a longer life. Poor heart health can lead to diseases that not only limit your quality of life but can also shorten it. It's understandable then, why taking control of your cardiovascular health is critical, especially as you age. This section of the book is dedicated to guiding you step-by-step on how to improve your heart health and, by extension, your overall well-being.

The first step in taking control is to recognize that you have the power to influence your health outcomes. Many factors that contribute to heart disease, such as diet, exercise, and stress management, are within your control. Acknowledging this is empowering and is the first step towards making lasting changes. We will explore each of these factors in detail, offering practical advice on how to integrate heart-healthy habits into your everyday life.

Let's begin with diet, a foundational aspect of heart health. What you eat directly impacts your cardiovascular system. Foods high in saturated fats, trans fats, and cholesterol can increase blood cholesterol levels, leading to plaque buildup in the arteries, which is a primary cause of heart disease. Conversely, a diet rich in fruits, vegetables, whole grains, and lean proteins can help reduce your risk. This is not just about avoiding bad foods but also about incorporating good ones that support heart health. We will delve into what specific foods to eat, how often, and in what quantities.

Next, we consider the role of exercise in maintaining a healthy heart. Physical activity helps improve heart function, lower blood pressure, and improve cholesterol levels and reverse diabetes. But how much exercise do you need? What types are most effective? These are important questions that we will address. You will receive clear guidelines on how to start an exercise regimen that fits your current fitness level and how to safely increase your activity over time.

Stress management is another critical area. Chronic stress can lead to high blood pressure, a risk factor for heart disease. In this section, we will talk about practical strategies for managing stress, such as mindfulness, meditation, and time management. These techniques can help reduce your stress levels and improve your heart health. Each method will be explained in simple terms, providing you with clear directions on how to incorporate these practices into your daily routine.

Beyond individual habits, it's also important to consider your overall lifestyle. This includes getting enough sleep, avoiding smoking, and managing your weight. Each of these lifestyle factors plays a crucial role in heart health. We will explore why these factors matter and provide you with straightforward strategies to improve each area. The importance of sleep cannot be overstated, as poor sleep has been linked to higher risk of heart disease. You will learn how to create a conducive sleeping environment and habits that promote restful sleep.

Finally, we will wrap up this section by putting it all together into a coherent plan that you can follow. This plan will include daily, weekly, and monthly goals that are both achievable and effective in improving your heart health. It will be a personalized plan, tailored to your specific needs and circumstances, which will make it more enjoyable and easier to stick with over the long term. By the end of this section, you will have a clear understanding of the steps you need to take to improve your cardiovascular health and a plan in place to achieve it.

Remember, the goal here is not just to inform you but to transform your approach to heart health. Each piece of advice is designed to be actionable and impactful, allowing you to make real changes that will lead to tangible improvements in your health. It's about empowering you to take control of your well-being through informed, deliberate actions.

By taking the information provided here and applying it consistently, you can significantly improve your heart health and overall well-being. This is not just about avoiding disease; it's about thriving. With the right knowledge and actions, you can enjoy a healthier, more vibrant life at any age.

So, take these steps seriously, integrate them into your life, and watch as your health transforms. You have the power to shape your health outcomes, and this section will guide you every step of the way. Let's embark on this journey together, with each step taking you closer to a healthier heart and a better life.

The Cardiovascular System

The cardiovascular system is a complex and essential part of your body. It includes your heart and all the blood vessels that run throughout your body. Let's delve into what this means and why it's important for you, especially if you are over the age of 40 and focused on improving your longevity and quality of life.

The heart, a muscular organ about the size of your fist, sits in the center of your chest slightly tilted to the left. Its main job is straightforward but vital: to pump blood throughout your body. This blood provides oxygen and nutrients to tissues and takes away waste products. Every day, your heart beats about 100,000 times, sending 2,000 gallons of blood surging through your body. This process is crucial because every cell in your body needs oxygen and nutrients to thrive.

Your blood vessels are the roadways that carry blood from your heart to every part of your body and back again. There are three main types of blood vessels: arteries, veins, and capillaries. Arteries carry oxygen-rich blood away from the heart to the tissues. Veins carry oxygen-poor blood back to the heart. Capillaries, tiny vessels between arteries and veins, exchange nutrients and waste between blood and tissues.

Understanding this system is the first step towards managing your cardiovascular health. It's the basis for everything from how you exercise, to what you eat, and even how you manage stress. All of these factors play a role in the health of your cardiovascular system.

Now, let's talk about common cardiovascular conditions and their effects. These conditions can significantly impact your health and lifestyle, especially as you grow older. The most common cardiovascular conditions include coronary artery disease, heart attack, and stroke. Coronary artery disease occurs when the arteries that supply blood to the heart muscle become hardened and narrowed due to the buildup of plaque. This can reduce blood flow to the heart and lead to a heart attack, which happens when the blood flow to a part of the heart is blocked long enough that part of the heart muscle is damaged or dies.

Stroke is another critical condition related to the cardiovascular system. It occurs when the blood supply to part of your brain is interrupted or reduced, preventing brain tissue from getting oxygen and nutrients. Brain cells begin to die in minutes. A stroke can cause lasting brain damage, long-term disability, or even death. Understanding these conditions is crucial because they directly affect how well you can live your life, especially in your later years.

Each of these conditions can be influenced by various factors, some within your control and some not. However, knowing about them is a powerful step in managing your health. It is important to recognize that while genetics play a role in cardiovascular health, many aspects of heart health are under your personal control, such as diet, exercise, and avoiding smoking.

By understanding the anatomy and function of your cardiovascular system, along with the common conditions that can affect it, you're better equipped to take steps towards preventing these conditions or managing them if they occur. It's all about providing your heart and blood vessels with what they need to do their job well, so you can continue to enjoy a life full of vitality and joy.

So, take this information to heart. Start considering how your lifestyle choices affect your cardiovascular health. Think about incorporating more physical activity into your day, choosing heart-healthy foods, and scheduling regular check-ups with your doctor. Each of these actions can make a significant difference in how well your cardiovascular system functions, helping you to lead a healthier, longer life.

This is just the beginning of understanding and taking charge of your cardiovascular health. By taking proactive steps now, you are paving the way for a healthier future, one where your heart continues to beat strongly, supporting you as you enjoy the best parts of life with those you love.

Risk Factors: Genetics and Lifestyle

When we talk about cardiovascular diseases, two major categories of factors affect our heart health: genetics and lifestyle. Understanding these can help us take proactive steps toward maintaining or improving our cardiovascular health.

Let's start by discussing genetics. Genes are like tiny instructions inside every cell of our body. They determine various characteristics, such as the color of our eyes, height, and even some health risks. In terms of heart health, some of us inherit genes from our parents that could increase our risk of cardiovascular diseases. These genetic factors can predispose us to high blood pressure, high cholesterol levels, and other heart-related issues. It's important to understand that inheriting such genes does not guarantee the development of cardiovascular conditions, but it does increase the likelihood compared to someone without these genetic traits.

While we cannot change our genetic makeup, being aware of our family's health history can prompt us to take early and more focused preventive measures. If you know that your family has a history of heart diseases, sharing this information with your healthcare provider can help tailor a monitoring and prevention plan that suits your specific needs. For example, regular screenings for blood pressure and cholesterol could be started earlier than typically recommended.

Now, let's shift our focus to lifestyle factors. These are the elements of our daily living that we can control and modify. Lifestyle factors include our diet, exercise habits, smoking status, alcohol consumption, and stress management, among others. Each of these factors plays a significant role in the condition of our cardiovascular health.

Diet is a cornerstone of heart health. Foods high in saturated fats, trans fats, and cholesterol can raise blood cholesterol levels, while a diet rich in fruits, vegetables, whole grains, and lean proteins can help reduce the risk of heart disease. Regular physical activity is equally important. It helps maintain a healthy weight, lowers blood pressure, and strengthens the heart. Just 150 minutes of moderate-intensity aerobic exercise per week can contribute greatly to cardiovascular health.

Smoking is a major risk factor for cardiovascular diseases. It damages the lining of the arteries and reduces the amount of oxygen that your blood can carry. Quitting smoking can significantly reduce the risk of developing heart diseases as well as other health issues. Alcohol, when consumed in excess, can lead to high blood pressure and other heart-related issues. However, moderate consumption might have some heart benefits, though this should always be discussed with a healthcare provider to ensure it fits within your personal health plan.

Stress management is another important aspect of a heart-healthy lifestyle. Chronic stress may lead to behaviors and factors that increase heart disease risk, such as high blood pressure and cholesterol levels, physical inactivity, and overeating. Finding healthy ways to manage stress, like regular exercise, adequate sleep, and relaxation techniques, can improve your overall health and reduce your cardiovascular risk.

Each of these lifestyle factors provides us with choices. Every positive choice we make can lead to a healthier heart and a reduced risk of heart disease. However, making changes can be challenging, especially if you are trying to change several habits at once. It is often more effective to focus on one or two changes at a time. Establishing new, healthier routines in place of old habits can take some time, but the benefits to heart health are worth the effort.

In summary, understanding both the genetic and lifestyle risk factors for cardiovascular disease empowers us to take charge of our heart health. While we cannot change our genetics, we can certainly influence our lifestyle choices. Regular consultations with healthcare providers, mindful eating, consistent physical activity, avoiding smoking, moderate alcohol consumption, and effective stress management can all constitute a robust defense against the onset of heart-related illnesses. By making informed choices, you can significantly enhance your longevity and quality of life.

Remember, the journey to better heart health is a continuous one. Each small step you take can lead to big improvements in your cardiovascular condition and overall well-being. Start today by evaluating your lifestyle choices and considering positive changes. Discussing your genetic background and lifestyle with healthcare professionals can also provide you with tailored strategies to effectively manage your heart health for years to come.

The Importance of Early Detection

Knowing about the presence of cardiovascular issues early can make a significant difference in how these conditions affect you long-term. It is crucial to spot warning signs and symptoms as soon as possible. Let's dive deeper into why this matters and which symptoms you should be on the lookout for.

Firstly, understanding the warning signs of cardiovascular issues is your first line of defense against serious health complications. Some common symptoms include chest pain, shortness of breath, excessive fatigue, and more. These might sound general, but they are critical indicators that something might be wrong with your heart or blood vessels.

If you experience any of these symptoms, it's important to consult a healthcare professional without delay. This step is not just about getting treatment but confirming whether these signs are indeed related to cardiovascular problems. Early detection can lead to early treatment, which significantly improves the outcome.

Moreover, regular check-ups play a pivotal role in catching cardiovascular diseases before they develop into severe conditions. During a check-up, your doctor can perform various screenings and tests that assess your heart health. These might include blood pressure measurements, cholesterol levels, and other key markers that indicate your cardiovascular health status.

Regular screenings are beneficial not only for detecting disease but also for monitoring the progress of existing conditions. If you are already diagnosed with a cardiovascular issue, these check-ups become even more crucial. They help your doctor make informed decisions about adjustments needed in your treatment plan.

Now, let's consider the benefits of these actions. Early detection through symptoms awareness and regular check-ups leads to early intervention. This early intervention is often less invasive and more effective. For example, managing high blood pressure with medication and lifestyle changes is simpler and cheaper than treating a heart attack, which might require surgery or other complex procedures.

Additionally, knowing you have a cardiovascular condition earlier rather than later gives you the valuable opportunity to adjust your lifestyle to better support your heart health. This might include dietary changes, increasing physical activity, quitting smoking, and other modifications that can have a profound impact on your overall well-being.

Prevention is always better than cure, and in the context of cardiovascular health, it is a mantra worth living by. Adopting a proactive approach towards your heart health can spare you from complications and enhance your quality of life significantly. It can also reduce medical costs in the long-run as preventive measures are typically less costly than treatments for advanced diseases.

In conclusion, the importance of early detection cannot be overstated. Recognizing the warning signs and symptoms of cardiovascular issues, coupled with regular health check-ups and screenings, are essential steps in preventing severe heart diseases. These practices empower you to take timely actions that can lead to better health outcomes. Make sure to consult with your healthcare provider about how often you should be screened based on your personal health history and risk factors. Taking these steps is not just about living longer; it's about living better.

Remember, your heart is the engine of your body. Just like any engine, it needs regular maintenance to run smoothly. Take care of your heart, and it will take care of you.

The Impact on Quality of Life

When we talk about cardiovascular diseases, we often focus on the medical aspects, symptoms, treatments, and prognosis. But the true measure of these diseases often lies in their profound impact on one's quality of life. Quality of life encompasses both physical and emotional dimensions, influencing daily activities, emotional well-being, and interpersonal relationships.

Physical limitations are one of the most visible effects of cardiovascular diseases. For instance, someone with heart disease may experience shortness of breath during activities that were once effortless. This can make walking, climbing stairs, or even carrying groceries challenging. The need to frequently rest can also disrupt daily routines, making it hard to maintain a normal work schedule or participate in social activities. This decreased physical capacity redefines a person's role within their family and community, sometimes leading to frustration and a diminished sense of self-worth.

Beyond the physical restrictions, the emotional challenges that come with cardiovascular diseases can be equally debilitating. It is not uncommon for individuals to experience feelings of anxiety and depression. The constant worry about health can overshadow the joy in everyday life. The stress of managing a chronic condition, coupled with fears of potential health crises, can strain even the strongest minds.

The family and community are also significantly affected by one individual's illness. Care responsibilities often fall on close family members, which can alter family dynamics and lead to stress in relationships. Social life can suffer, too, as social interactions often decrease. Friends and community members might not understand the full extent of the disease's impact, leading to feelings of isolation for the person affected.

Understanding the broad impact of cardiovascular diseases on quality of life is crucial. Acknowledging these challenges is the first step toward managing them effectively. By addressing both the physical and emotional sides of these diseases, individuals and families can work towards maintaining a fulfilling life despite the diagnosis. This includes seeking not only medical help but also emotional and social support.

The next sections will explore how to address these challenges practically and empathetically, ensuring that people dealing with cardiovascular diseases can lead as rich and fulfilling a life as possible. It is possible to manage the disease with proper care and support, and to continue living a life that is not only about survival but also about well-being and happiness.

Current Research and Statistics

The world of cardiovascular health is always evolving. Every year, researchers across the globe are working tirelessly to uncover new findings that can help us manage and prevent heart diseases. What have they discovered recently? Let's dive into the latest research and statistics.

Firstly, it's important to understand that cardiovascular disease remains one of the leading causes of death worldwide, despite advances in medical technology and knowledge. This fact alone emphasizes the need for ongoing research and innovation in this field. With each study, doctors and scientists gather more data, helping to refine treatment plans and prevention strategies.

Recent studies have shown a promising link between lifestyle modifications and the reduction of heart disease risk. For example, research indicates that regular physical activity can reduce the risk of developing heart-related issues by up to 25%. It is a simple yet effective way to strengthen the heart and improve blood circulation. Regular exercise helps maintain a healthy weight, which is crucial because obesity is a significant risk factor for cardiovascular disease.

Another critical area of recent research focuses on dietary impacts on heart health. Studies consistently show the benefits of a diet rich in fruits, vegetables, lean proteins, and whole grains. Researchers have found that diets low in saturated fats and high in fiber can lead to better cardiovascular outcomes. Moreover, reducing salt intake has been linked to lower blood pressure levels, which is a major risk factor for stroke and heart attack.

Statistics also play a crucial role in understanding the scope of cardiovascular health challenges. Data from health organizations show trends and projections that are essential for public health planning. For instance, it has been projected that by 2030, almost 23.6 million people will die annually from cardiovascular diseases. This projection highlights the urgent need for intensified research and preventive measures.

Additionally, advancements in technology offer new ways to manage heart health. Wearable technology that monitors heart rate, blood pressure, and even blood sugar levels can provide real-time data for users and their healthcare providers. This technology enables more personalized and immediate adjustments to treatment plans.

It's also worth noting that the field of genetics has brought new insights into cardiovascular diseases. Research has identified specific genetic markers associated with increased risk of heart disease, leading to the development of genetic screening tools. With these tools, individuals can be aware of their predisposition to heart issues early on, allowing for preventive measures to be implemented sooner rather than later.

Despite these advancements, challenges remain. Access to healthcare, socioeconomic factors, and global disparities in health education continue to impact cardiovascular disease rates negatively.

Addressing these issues requires a combined effort from governments, health organizations, and individuals alike.

To wrap up, staying informed about the latest research and statistics in cardiovascular health is crucial. It not only helps individuals make informed decisions about their health but also guides policymakers in creating effective health interventions. By understanding and utilizing current data, we can all contribute to a heart-healthier future.

Remember, every step you take towards understanding and applying the latest research in your daily life can significantly impact your cardiovascular health. Whether it's adopting a healthier diet, integrating regular exercise into your routine, or keeping up with regular check-ups, these actions are valuable. They are not just statistics; they are lives saved, enhanced health, and improved quality of life.

So, take this information and use it. Adjust your lifestyle, consult with healthcare professionals, and take advantage of the technology and resources available to you. Together, let's work towards a future where cardiovascular disease is no longer a leading cause of death, but a manageable and preventable condition.

Chapter Recap

So far, we have learned a lot about cardiovascular disease and its importance in our lives, especially as we grow older. Let's take a moment to go over some of the key points we've discussed. This will not only help in reinforcing what we've learned but will also make it easier for you to see what steps you can take next.

Firstly, we explored the cardiovascular system, comprising the heart and the blood vessels. This system is crucial as it transports nutrients, oxygen, and hormones to cells throughout the body and removes metabolic wastes. Problems here can lead to significant health issues, so understanding it is the first step in taking better care of our heart health.

We then looked into the risk factors that can affect our cardiovascular health. Some factors, like genetics, are beyond our control, which emphasizes the importance of managing the factors we can control such as diet, exercise, and smoking habits.

Early detection of cardiovascular issues was another critical topic we covered. Knowing the warning signs and symptoms can make a significant difference in managing health outcomes. Regular check-ups and screenings are not something to put off, as they can potentially save your life by catching problems before they become severe.

The impact of cardiovascular diseases on quality of life cannot be understated. Both physical limitations and emotional struggles can arise, affecting not just the individual but also their families and communities. It's essential to address these challenges holistically, considering both medical and emotional support.

Finally, we discussed the latest research and statistics which help us understand the trends in cardiovascular health. This knowledge empowers us to make informed decisions about our health management strategies.

Now, it's time to turn this knowledge into action. Here are some specific steps you can take:

- **Assess Your Personal Risk Factors:** Start by looking at your family history. Does heart disease run in your family? Next, evaluate your lifestyle. Are you getting enough exercise? What's your diet like? Do you smoke? Addressing these questions can help you identify areas where you can reduce your risk.
- **Schedule Regular Check-Ups:** If you haven't seen a doctor in a while, now is the time to schedule a check-up. Regular screenings for blood pressure, cholesterol, and other markers can help catch problems early.
- **Adjust Your Diet:** Incorporate heart-healthy foods into your diet. Focus on eating plenty of fruits, vegetables, whole grains, and lean proteins. Reduce intake of salts, fats, and sugars. Remember, small changes can lead to big benefits over time.
- **Increase Physical Activity:** Aim for at least 150 minutes of moderate aerobic exercise or 75 minutes of vigorous exercise each week. Activities like walking, cycling, or swimming can make a significant difference in your heart health.
- **Manage Stress:** Chronic stress can contribute to heart disease. Find stress management techniques that work for you, such as meditation, yoga, or spending time on hobbies you love.

Remember, the goal is not just to live longer but to enjoy a higher quality of life. By taking these steps, you're not only improving your heart health but also investing in a future where you can remain active and engaged with your loved ones and life itself. It's never too late to start making changes, and every small step counts.

As we move forward, keep these points in mind. Refer back to them as you make health and lifestyle decisions. Heart health is a lifelong commitment, and you have the power to influence your future. Let's embrace this journey with knowledge, action, and optimism.

Thank you for taking this time to focus on your cardiovascular health. By understanding and addressing these issues proactively, you're setting yourself on a path towards a healthier and more fulfilling life.

What is Intermittent Fasting?

Introduction to Intermittent Fasting

Intermittent fasting is a method of scheduling meals during specific times to achieve and maintain good health, especially as you age. It is not just about choosing what to eat but also when to eat. This approach focuses on the timing of meals, allowing for regular periods of eating intermixed with periods of fasting. The primary idea here is not to cut calories drastically but to allocate your eating to certain time windows throughout the day.

The concept is straightforward: you switch between periods of eating and fasting. This could mean eating only during an eight-hour window each day and fasting for the remaining 16 hours. Another common approach is the 5:2 method, where you eat normally for five days of the week and limit your calorie intake on the other two days.

One of the key principles of intermittent fasting is its flexibility and adaptability to different lifestyles and health needs. It is not a one-size-fits-all answer but a customizable approach that can accommodate varied dietary habits and routines.

There are multiple ways to implement this eating pattern. Some people prefer daily time-restricted feeding windows, while others find success in fasting for whole days one or two times a week. Let's explore these methods in more detail to understand how they could be beneficial.

Daily Time-Restricted Feeding: This method involves eating all meals within a designated 6-8 hour period each day, often skipping breakfast and making lunch the first meal of the day. The fasting period includes the time spent sleeping overnight, effectively extending the fasting window without additional effort.

The 5:2 Diet: In this approach, you eat normally for five days of the week but restrict calories to about 500-600 for the other two days, which do not have to be consecutive. This method reduces weekly calorie intake without requiring constant calorie counting or changing what you eat significantly.

24-Hour Fasts: This technique, also known as the eat-stop-eat method, involves fasting for 24 hours once or twice a week. This could mean not eating from dinner one day until dinner the next day. It's a more advanced method that may be suitable for those who have experience with shorter fasts.

Alternate-Day Fasting: This involves alternating days of no food restriction with days where food intake is severely limited to about 500 calories. This method might be challenging to maintain but can be effective for significant weight loss and health improvement.

The variety in these methods allows you to choose the one that best fits your lifestyle, preferences, and health goals. It is essential, however, to select a method that you can sustain over the long term as intermittent fasting is not just a diet but a lifestyle change.

When you fast, several things happen in your body on the

cellular and molecular level. For example, your body adjusts hormone levels to make stored body fat more accessible. Your cells also initiate important repair processes and change the expression of genes. These changes are part of why intermittent fasting can help manage weight and improve metabolic health, which are crucial as you grow older.

It's important to approach intermittent fasting with a mindset focused on health rather than just weight loss. Think of it as a way to reset your body's internal clock, not just a tool to reduce calories. When done correctly, intermittent fasting can lead to improved heart health, better blood sugar control, reduced inflammation, and increased longevity.

To start with intermittent fasting, choose a method that seems manageable for you and start slowly. For instance, begin with a shorter fasting window and gradually increase the duration as your body adjusts. It's also vital to maintain a balanced diet during your eating periods; fasting does not compensate for bad eating habits.

Choose whole foods rather than ultraprocessed foods. Ultraprocessed foods will spike insulin which causes weight gain. Hormonal weight gain is very common way to gain weight and cause cardiovascular diseases. Even if you eat less of the wrong food like junck food, you get hungry sooner because the food goes strait into storage. Best way to lower the hormone insulin is to fast. Intermittent fasting is a period of time when you dont eat letting your insulin to drop. This is best achieved not eating for 16 hours at least.

Lastly, consult with a healthcare provider before starting any new dietary regimen, especially if you have underlying health conditions or are on medication. Intermittent fasting offers many benefits, but it is crucial to ensure it's a safe option for your specific health needs.

Understanding and implementing intermittent fasting can be a step toward better cardiovascular health and overall wellness. This method helps not only in managing weight but also in stabilizing blood sugar levels, reducing inflammation, and improving heart health. As you move through your 40s and beyond, these health markers become increasingly important in maintaining a high quality of life.

Adopting intermittent fasting into your lifestyle could be a transformative experience, but it should be approached with care, consideration, and professional guidance. With the right approach, it can be an effective tool to enhance your health and longevity.

The Science Behind Fasting

When you choose to fast, your body undergoes significant changes. These changes impact how your body functions and can have profound effects on your health, particularly your heart health. Understanding these changes is essential if you are looking to use fasting as a tool to enhance your cardiovascular health.

The first change occurs at the physiological level. Initially, your body uses glucose stored in the liver and muscles as its primary source of energy. This glucose is stored in a form called glycogen. During the first few hours of fasting, your body breaks down this glycogen into glucose. It's like your body has a reserve fuel tank that it starts to use once the regular supply is cut off.

Once the glycogen stores are depleted, which usually happens after about 12 to 16 hours of fasting, your body needs to find a new source of energy. This is where the fat reserves come into play. The body begins a process called ketosis. In ketosis, fat is converted into fatty acids and ketone bodies. These ketone bodies then become the main energy source for your body and brain. This shift from using glucose to using fat as a fuel is a significant transition and central to the benefits of fasting.

During this metabolic shift, several hormonal changes also occur. One of the primary hormones affected is insulin. Insulin levels drop significantly when you fast, which facilitates fat burning. Lower insulin levels combined with increased levels of the hormone glucagon lead to increased fat breakdown. It's a natural response that helps your body to continue functioning without its usual intake of food.

Another hormone that fasting affects is human growth hormone (HGH). Levels of HGH can skyrocket during a fast, increasing as much as five-fold. This increase in HGH not only helps in fat loss but also in muscle gain and other restorative body processes. This hormone plays a significant role in health, fitness, and slowing the aging process.

Norepinephrine is another hormone that fasting boosts. This hormone is linked to alertness and energy. It's one of the reasons why many people report feeling more energetic during fasting periods, despite not eating. Your body releases norepinephrine to help you stay active and alert while you're not consuming food. It is as if your body is making sure you are ready to be on the move, should you need to find food in a natural scarcity scenario.

The metabolic switch to ketosis, along with changes in hormones like insulin, glucagon, human growth hormone, and norepinephrine, all contribute to why fasting can be such a powerful method for improving health. These physiological and hormonal changes lead to numerous benefits, such as improved metabolism, better brain function, increased fat burning, and decreased inflammation. These changes are closely linked to improved cardiovascular health, which is crucial for anyone looking to enhance their longevity and quality of life, especially adults over 40.

It's also worth noting the impact of fasting on inflammation and oxidative stress, two factors closely linked to heart disease. Studies have shown that fasting can decrease markers of inflammation and reduce oxidative damage. Oxidative stress is essentially an imbalance between free radicals and antioxidants in your body. Free radicals are oxygen-containing molecules with an uneven number of electrons, which allows them to easily react with other molecules. These reactions can cause large chain chemical reactions in your body because they react so easily with other molecules. These reactions are called oxidation. They can be harmful when they happen in excess, damaging cells and body structures, including blood vessels, which can lead to heart disease.

Reducing oxidative stress and inflammation can therefore be particularly beneficial for heart health. By fasting, you're not only helping your heart to manage its current workloads better but also preventing future heart disease by taking care of these underlying biological mechanisms.

Fasting is not just about reducing calorie intake but about initiating a complex, beneficial series of events in your body. By understanding and harnessing these physiological and hormonal changes, fasting can be a powerful tool to enhance your overall health and protect your cardiovascular system. It is an actionable, natural, and effective method to help manage and prevent heart diseases, especially for those over the age of 40 who are looking to improve their longevity and quality of life.

Fasting and Cardiovascular Health

When people think about fasting, they often focus on its role in weight loss or detoxification. However, there's a significant area where fasting plays a crucial role, and that's in the maintenance and improvement of cardiovascular health. Cardiovascular diseases, which include heart attacks, stroke, and heart failure, are a leading cause of death globally. Given this, finding effective strategies to prevent or manage these diseases is paramount, especially as we age.

One of the ways fasting benefits cardiovascular health is through its impact on various heart health markers. These markers are specific indicators in your body that can provide information about your heart's health. Some of these markers include blood pressure, levels of various types of cholesterol, and blood sugar levels. Managing these markers can significantly reduce the risk of cardiovascular diseases. Fasting has been shown to influence these markers positively, but how does this happen? Let's delve deeper into this topic.

The answer lies in the body's physiological response to the fasting state. When you fast, your body undergoes several changes at the hormonal and metabolic levels, which we've touched on briefly in the previous sections. For cardiovascular health specifically, fasting improves metabolic efficiency and lowers metabolic risks associated with heart disease. For example, fasting can lead to reductions in blood pressure. High blood pressure is a significant risk factor for heart disease as it forces the heart to work harder to pump blood, which can weaken the heart over time and contribute to plaque build-up in the arteries.

Furthermore, fasting influences cholesterol levels. It typically lowers the levels of LDL cholesterol, often referred to as 'bad' cholesterol. LDL cholesterol is known for contributing to the buildup of plaques in the arteries, which can lead to atherosclerosis, a condition that can cause heart attacks and stroke. By reducing the levels of LDL cholesterol, fasting helps keep the arteries clear and reduces the risk of heart disease.

Additionally, fasting can help regulate blood sugar levels, which is particularly important for preventing or managing diabetes, a known risk factor for cardiovascular diseases. During fasting, as the body runs low on its immediate glucose supply, it starts converting fat into energy. This process not only aids in weight management but also helps stabilize blood sugar levels over time.

But how does fasting trigger these beneficial changes? The mechanics can be attributed to a process known as autophagy. Autophagy is the body's way of cleaning out damaged cells, in order to regenerate newer, healthier cells. During fasting, the rates of autophagy are increased. This process is beneficial for the heart as it involves the removal of dysfunctional proteins and cellular debris from cells, which can prevent diseases like heart disease and diabetes.

Moreover, fasting has an anti-inflammatory effect on the body. Chronic inflammation is associated with an increased risk of heart disease, among other health issues. By lowering the inflammation levels in the body, fasting can thus play a role in reducing the risk of heart complications.

Given these points, it’s clear that intermittent fasting can be a powerful tool in the prevention and management of cardiovascular diseases. By understanding these mechanisms, you can better appreciate why adopting fasting could be beneficial. However, it is essential to approach this practice correctly.

Fasting should be done under the guidance of a healthcare professional, especially if you have pre-existing health conditions or are on medication. It's also crucial to choose a method of fasting that fits well with your lifestyle and health needs. There are various fasting methods, such as the 16/8 method, where you eat during an eight-hour window and fast for 16 hours, or the 5:2 method, where you eat regularly for five days and reduce your calorie intake significantly for the other two days of the week.

To integrate fasting into your life effectively, start slowly and monitor how your body reacts. It is also essential to maintain a balanced diet during your eating periods. Ensuring you consume nutrient-dense foods will support your body's needs and enhance the health benefits of fasting. Remember, the goal is to improve your health, so taking a balanced and informed approach is key.

In conclusion, fasting offers several mechanisms that benefit heart health, from lowering blood pressure and cholesterol to reducing blood sugar levels and inflammation. By understanding these mechanisms and carefully integrating fasting into your lifestyle with professional guidance, you can harness these benefits to improve your cardiovascular health significantly. This approach not only helps in managing existing conditions but also in preventing the onset of cardiovascular diseases, leading to a healthier, more vibrant life.

Success Stories and Case Studies

When we talk about improving heart health through intermittent fasting, real-life examples can provide the encouragement and evidence needed to take the first step. Many adults over 40 have turned to intermittent fasting not just to lose weight but to enhance their cardiovascular health. It's essential to understand that each journey is unique, and while the outcomes might vary, the overarching theme is positive change.

Consider the story of John, a 52-year-old man who was diagnosed with borderline high blood pressure and cholesterol. Concerned about his heart health, he decided to try intermittent fasting after hearing about its benefits from his doctor. John opted for the 16/8 method, where he ate all his meals within an 8-hour window and fasted for the remaining 16 hours of the day. Over the months, not only did he lose excess weight, but his blood pressure and cholesterol levels improved significantly. His doctor was pleased with his progress, noting that John's risk of cardiovascular diseases had decreased.

Then there's Maria, a 47-year-old woman who struggled with obesity and was at risk for heart disease. Maria chose a 5:2 intermittent fasting plan, eating normally for five days and significantly reducing her calorie intake for two days of the week. This not only helped her manage her weight but also led to better regulation of her blood sugar levels, a vital factor in cardiovascular health. After a year of intermittent fasting, Maria reported feeling more energetic, and her heart health markers had stabilized into a healthier range.

Stories like John's and Maria's highlight the potential of intermittent fasting to transform health. It's important to note that they both consulted their healthcare providers before starting. They were monitored throughout their journey to ensure the changes in diet and routine were beneficial and not detrimental to their health.

These case studies serve as a motivational tool and a blueprint for others considering similar health transformations. They show that with the right method, consistent effort, and medical guidance, significant improvements in cardiovascular health are achievable. More so, they emphasize the importance of personalized approaches in health and wellness.

Seeing real-life examples helps demystify the process and outcomes of intermittent fasting for heart health. It changes the narrative from a daunting challenge to a manageable and rewarding endeavor. It also illustrates the importance of being proactive about health. John and Maria didn't wait for severe health problems to take action. Instead, they took control of their health trajectories, paving the way for a healthier future.

These stories reinforce the concept that while intermittent fasting can be highly beneficial, it is not a magic bullet. It requires careful planning, consultation with healthcare providers, and a commitment to long-term lifestyle changes. But as seen through the experiences of real people, the results can be profoundly impactful, leading not only to better cardiovascular health but also to improved overall well-being.

In conclusion, the success stories of individuals who have embraced intermittent fasting for heart health serve as powerful testimonials to its potential benefits. These narratives not only inspire but also provide practical frameworks that others can adapt to their situations. They remind us that taking small, calculated steps towards improving our diet and fasting routines can lead to significant health benefits, particularly in preventing and managing cardiovascular diseases.

Addressing Concerns and Misconceptions

When we talk about intermittent fasting, some people feel uneasy. They have heard things that make them worry. Maybe they think fasting is not safe or that it could hurt their health. Today, we'll look at these worries and clear up any misunderstandings about intermittent fasting, especially for those concerned about cardiovascular health.

One common concern is that fasting might cause muscle loss. It's a valid worry. No one wants to lose muscle instead of fat. But the truth is, if done properly, intermittent fasting targets fat more than muscle. Our bodies are smart. When fasting, our body shifts to using stored fat for energy, preserving muscle mass. However, it is crucial to follow a well-planned fasting schedule and eat nutritious foods during your eating periods to support muscle health.

Another worry people have is about feeling weak or dizzy during fasting. This can happen, especially when starting a fasting routine. Our bodies need time to adjust. Starting with shorter fasting periods and gradually increasing the duration can help your body adapt. Also, staying hydrated is essential. Many times, feelings of weakness are actually signs of dehydration, not lack of food.

Heart health is a big concern for many, especially those over 40. Some fear that fasting could stress the heart. Let's address this: research indicates that intermittent fasting may actually improve heart health by reducing blood pressure, inflammation, and blood sugar levels. These factors are closely linked to heart disease. Of course, if you have existing heart conditions or concerns, talking to a doctor before starting any new diet, including intermittent fasting, is a good step. Medical supervision ensures your approach is tailored to your personal health needs.

People also worry about the drop in energy levels. It's true, during the first few days of intermittent fasting, you might feel less energetic. This is part of the adjustment period. But many report higher energy levels and increased alertness once they adapt to the fasting routine. It's like resetting your body's energy usage. It starts to run more efficiently on its fat stores.

Let's also talk about the concern that fasting is just another diet fad. Intermittent fasting is based on research, not just trends. Historical evidence shows that fasting has been a part of human culture and health practices for millennia. Modern science now explains why it can be beneficial, showing how it affects metabolism, aging, and cellular repair processes. It's not about quick fixes but about making a sustainable change in how and when you eat.

Lastly, there is often a concern about the difficulty of sticking to a fasting schedule. This is a real challenge. Life is unpredictable, and finding a consistent time to eat and fast can be tough. However, intermittent fasting offers flexibility. There are various approaches, such as the 16/8 method or 5:2 method, which can fit different lifestyles and preferences. It’s about finding what works for you, making it easier to maintain in the long term.

In conclusion, while concerns about intermittent fasting are understandable, most are based on misconceptions or incomplete information. With proper planning, adaptation, and medical advice when needed, intermittent fasting can be a safe, effective way to improve health and protect your heart. Always remember to listen to your body and consult healthcare professionals to tailor fasting and dietary practices that best suit your health needs and lifestyle.

Embracing a new eating pattern can be a significant change, but it's also a chance to take charge of your health. By addressing these concerns and providing clear, factual information, we hope you feel more confident and informed about how intermittent fasting might fit into your lifestyle, particularly in supporting your cardiovascular health as you age.

Chapter Recap

As we wrap up this chapter on the power of intermittent fasting, it's crucial to solidify the key points we've covered and understand how you can apply them to improve your cardiovascular health. This chapter has provided a deep dive into what intermittent fasting is, the scientific mechanisms behind it, its direct benefits on heart health, and addressed common concerns and misconceptions. Now, let's summarize these insights and outline specific steps you can take to integrate intermittent fasting into your lifestyle.

Intermittent fasting involves alternating periods of eating with periods of not eating. This practice isn't just about skipping meals; it's a structured approach to reducing your eating windows, which can significantly affect your body's physiological processes. The benefits range from hormone regulation, like increasing insulin sensitivity, to enhancing heart function by improving blood pressure and reducing inflammation.

One of the reasons intermittent fasting is beneficial for heart health is its ability to prompt physiological changes that favor heart health. For instance, fasting can lead to improved blood lipid profiles, including reductions in LDL cholesterol and triglycerides, which are crucial for preventing cardiovascular diseases. Moreover, fasting has been shown to enhance autophagy, the process by which your body cleans out damaged cells, which can help in preventing plaque buildup in your arteries.

Despite its benefits, intermittent fasting can seem daunting due to prevalent myths and misconceptions. It is often thought that fasting can lead to extreme hunger or loss of muscle mass. However, these effects are generally minimal, especially when the fasting period is well-planned and includes nutrient-rich foods during eating windows.

Now that you understand the basics and the benefits of intermittent fasting, as well as the reassurances against common fears, it's time to consider how you can start incorporating this practice into your life. Here are some actionable steps:

- **Choose a Fasting Method:** There are several methods of intermittent fasting, each with different eating and fasting windows. Some popular methods include the 16/8 method, where you fast for 16 hours and eat during an 8-hour window, or the 5:2 method, where you consume a regular diet five days a week and limit your calorie intake for the remaining two days. Evaluate your daily routine and choose a method that you feel you can adhere to consistently.
- **Start Gradually:** If you're new to intermittent fasting, it's wise to start slowly. Begin by delaying breakfast or moving up your dinner time to shorten your eating window gradually. This gradual adaptation can help your body adjust without significant stress.
- **Monitor Your Body's Response:** Pay attention to how your body responds during the fasting periods. Common initial reactions include hunger and irritability, but these usually decrease as your body adapts. If you experience severe adverse effects, reconsider the fasting plan or consult a healthcare professional.
- **Focus on Nutrient-Dense Foods:** During your eating windows, focus on consuming foods rich in nutrients, fruits, vegetables, lean

proteins, and whole grains. Avoid the temptation to indulge in unhealthy foods just because the eating window is limited.

- **Stay Hydrated:** Drinking plenty of water is essential during fasting periods. Water helps stave off hunger and maintains hydration, crucial for overall health and particularly vital when you are not consuming food regularly.
- **Consult Your Healthcare Provider:** Before starting any new dietary regimen, particularly if you have existing health conditions or are taking medication, it is crucial to consult with your healthcare provider. They can provide guidance tailored to your health needs and ensure your fasting method is safe and effective.

By following these steps, you can begin to integrate intermittent fasting into your routine in a safe, effective way that supports your cardiovascular health. Remember, the goal is not just to adopt a new diet but to embrace a sustainable lifestyle change that can significantly enhance your quality of life and longevity.

As you embark on this journey, keep track of your progress and be patient with yourself. Lifestyle changes take time to adjust, and gradual improvements are often more sustainable. With the right approach, intermittent fasting can be a powerful tool in your arsenal for heart health and overall well-being.

In conclusion, intermittent fasting offers a promising path for those looking to enhance their cardiovascular health and manage or prevent heart-related conditions. By understanding the principles, benefits, and methods of intermittent fasting, you can make informed decisions about incorporating this practice into your life. Follow the steps outlined above, consult professionals when necessary, and adopt a patient, persistent approach to reap the maximum benefits of intermittent fasting for your heart health.

Designing Your Fasting Plan

Assessing Your Lifestyle and Preferences

When you decide to start a fasting plan, the very first step is to look closely at your current lifestyle and preferences. This includes your work schedule, family obligations, and personal routines. Understanding these areas is fundamental because they greatly influence how successfully you can integrate fasting into your daily life.

Let's begin by examining your work schedule. Ask yourself, what hours do you work? Are you in a job that has fixed times, or is it flexible? For instance, someone who works a standard nine-to-five job might find it easier to plan meals around regular hours, whereas a shift worker might need a more adaptable fasting schedule.

Next, consider your family obligations. Do you have children who need meals at specific times? Are you responsible for preparing meals for others in your household? Your fasting plan needs to accommodate these responsibilities, ensuring that your commitment to fasting does not disrupt the dietary needs or routines of your family members.

Your personal routines also play a crucial role. Reflect on your current eating habits and preferences. Do you prefer a hearty breakfast, or do you usually skip it? Understanding your natural inclinations towards food will help you choose a fasting schedule that feels more natural and sustainable.

Now, let's talk about personal challenges and opportunities. Every individual faces unique challenges when adjusting to a new eating plan. For example, you might find it difficult to attend social gatherings without partaking in the meal. On the other hand, you might discover opportunities, such as a supportive partner who wants to join you on your fasting journey, which could make the process more enjoyable and feasible.

Identifying these challenges and opportunities requires honest self-reflection. It involves recognizing the hurdles that might come your way and preparing strategies to overcome them. Similarly, spotting opportunities where you can leverage support or integrate fasting more smoothly into your lifestyle will facilitate success.

Consider keeping a diary for a week to closely log your daily activities, eating habits, and how you feel throughout the day. This record can provide invaluable insights into the best way to tailor a fasting plan that aligns well with your lifestyle.

In conclusion, a thorough assessment of your current lifestyle and preferences is not just helpful; it is essential. It allows you to create a fasting plan that respects your personal life demands, tackles foreseeable challenges head-on, and uses every available opportunity to your advantage. With this thoughtful preparation, you set yourself up for a smoother and more effective fasting experience that can significantly aid in managing or preventing cardiovascular diseases, thereby enhancing your longevity and quality of life.

Remember, the goal is not just to start fasting but to integrate it seamlessly into your life so that it becomes a sustainable and beneficial part of your health routine. With the right plan that respects your personal circumstances, intermittent fasting can be a powerful tool in your health arsenal.

Choosing the Right Fasting Protocol

When it comes to improving cardiovascular health and enhancing longevity, selecting an appropriate fasting protocol is crucial. This decision will largely depend on understanding the various fasting methods available and finding one that aligns with your lifestyle.

Fasting methods such as the 16/8 method or the 5:2 diet have gained popularity due to their simplicity and effectiveness. The 16/8 method involves fasting for 16 hours each day and eating within an 8-hour window. This pattern can be easily adapted to fit daily schedules, especially for those who prefer not eating late in the evening or love having breakfast later in the day.

On the other hand, the 5:2 diet involves eating normally for five days of the week, while restricting calorie intake on the other two days to about 500-600 calories. This method is sometimes favored by individuals who find daily fasting to be challenging but can manage two days of reduced calorie intake without much trouble.

Deciding between these fasting strategies, or others like

alternate-day fasting or 24-hour fasts, requires consideration of your personal habits, work schedule, family commitments, and social life. Sustainability is key. You need a plan that feels less like a temporary diet and more like a manageable part of your everyday life.

To make a well-informed decision, start by evaluating your typical day. If your mornings are hectic, a fasting plan that skips breakfast but includes lunch and dinner might work best. Conversely, if evenings are your key time for socializing or family meals, a plan that allows for a hearty breakfast and lunch might be preferable, ending your eating window mid-afternoon.

Additionally, think about your capacity for handling hunger. If the idea of going long periods without food seems daunting, starting with a milder approach like the 12/12 method, fasting for 12 hours and eating within a 12-hour window, might ease you into the practice of fasting without overwhelming you.

It's also essential to consider your health status. For instance, if you have diabetes or other metabolic health conditions, you should consult with a healthcare provider before starting any fasting regimen. They can help tailor a fasting schedule that won't jeopardize your health and will complement any medical treatments you're currently undergoing.

Once you have thought about these factors, try starting with a less restrictive fasting method to see how your body responds. It's perfectly okay to adjust your fasting schedule as you go along. What works well for one person might not be ideal for another. The goal is to find a rhythm that contributes positively to your overall well-being and can be sustained over the long term.

Adjustments are part of the process. You might find that what starts as a 16/8 fasting schedule becomes a 14/10 schedule that better suits your lifestyle needs and health goals. The flexibility to tweak your fasting plan is crucial as it must evolve with your life's demands and changes.

Remember, the objective here is not just weight loss, though that can be a beneficial side effect, but overall cardiovascular health improvement. This means the fasting protocol you choose should not only be effective but should also feel right for you, integrating seamlessly into your daily life and enhancing your quality of life without adding undue stress or complexity.

In conclusion, think of choosing a fasting protocol not as a one-time decision but as a foundational element of a longer health journey. It's about experimenting responsibly, listening to your body, and adjusting accordingly. With the right approach, intermittent fasting can be a powerful tool in your arsenal for heart health and longevity, tailored specifically to suit your lifestyle and needs.

Planning Your Meals and Nutrition

When you decide to incorporate fasting into your lifestyle, one critical aspect to carefully plan is your meal and nutrition intake during your eating windows. The goal here is not just to eat, but to nourish your body with balanced, nutrient-dense foods that support heart health and overall well-being. This section will guide you through the process of selecting the right foods and planning your meals to ensure you derive the maximum benefit from your fasting regimen.

Firstly, understanding what 'nutrient-dense' foods mean is crucial. These are foods that have high nutrient content relative to their calorie content. They provide vitamins, minerals, complex carbohydrates, lean protein, and healthy fats. They do much more for your body than just satisfy hunger. For adults over 40, focusing on heart health, these nutrients play pivotal roles in maintaining and improving cardiovascular function.

When planning your meals, think about including a variety of foods from all the food groups. This diversity ensures that you receive a broad spectrum of nutrients essential for your body. Start with vegetables and fruits, which should take up half of your plate. They are rich in dietary fiber, vitamins, and minerals, all beneficial for heart health and help in managing body weight.

Next, consider your protein sources. Lean meats like chicken, turkey, and fish are excellent choices. Fish, particularly fatty types like salmon and mackerel, are high in omega-3 fatty acids, which are known to reduce inflammation and improve heart health. Plant-based proteins such as beans, lentils, and tofu are not only good protein sources but also bring additional fiber and minerals to your meals.

Whole grains form another crucial component of a heart-healthy diet. Options like whole wheat, brown rice, oats, and quinoa are excellent. They provide the necessary complex carbohydrates that give energy, are rich in fiber, and help in cholesterol management. Integrating these into your meals can be simple, like choosing whole-grain bread for sandwiches or using quinoa in salads.

Healthy fats are also essential, despite the common misconception that fats are bad for health. The key is choosing the right types of fats. Avocados, nuts, seeds, and olive oil are sources of healthy fats. These fats help absorb vitamins and provide essential fatty acids that your body cannot produce on its own. Including a small portion of healthy fats in your meals can aid in long-term heart health.

Hydration is another aspect you should not overlook. Water plays multiple roles in your body, including aiding digestion and maintaining blood pressure levels. Ensure you drink adequate amounts of water throughout the day, not just during your eating windows.

When it comes to putting all these elements together, planning is your best tool. Prepare a meal plan that covers various nutrients over different meals. This doesn't just help in adhering to a healthy diet; it also takes the guesswork out of what to eat during your eating window, making it less likely that you'll opt for convenient but unhealthy options.

Here are some tips to help you eat healthily during your eating windows:

1. Prepare in advance: Meal prep can save time and stress. Cook

large batches of dishes that align with your nutritional goals and use them throughout the week.

2. Focus on whole foods: Minimize the intake of processed foods, which often contain high levels of sodium, sugars, and unhealthy fats. These can negatively impact your cardiovascular health.

3. Monitor portion sizes: It's easy to overeat, even healthy foods, when you have fewer meals. Use smaller plates, bowls, and cups to help control portions.

4. Be mindful of eating: Pay attention to what and how much you eat. This practice helps to enjoy meals and recognize when you are full, reducing the chances of overeating.

5. Diversify your diet: Try new foods and recipes to keep your meals exciting and nutritionally diverse. This not only improves your nutrient intake but also makes adhering to a healthy diet more enjoyable.

By focusing on nutrient-rich foods and planning your meals wisely, you can significantly enhance the health benefits of your fasting plan. This approach not only helps in managing or preventing cardiovascular diseases but also supports overall health, ensuring you enjoy a higher quality of life as you age.

Remember, the key to successful meal planning during fasting is not just about restricting when you eat but about consciously deciding what you eat in your eating windows. This strategic approach ensures you get enough nutrients to support your body's needs, thereby maximizing the benefits of your fasting regimen. By following the guidelines provided, you will be better equipped to make informed and effective dietary choices that support your cardiovascular health and general well-being.

Allowing for Flexibility and Adjustments

When you embark on a journey to improve your health through fasting, understanding that flexibility is key can be very empowering. Life comes with its complexities. There are social events, family gatherings, unexpected travel, and simply days when your body doesn't feel aligned with your fasting schedule. Here, we will delve into practical strategies for maintaining your fasting regimen while accommodating the unpredictable nature of everyday life.

First and foremost, it's important to recognize that flexibility in your fasting plan doesn't mean you are deviating from your goals. It means you are adapting to ensure sustainability. Imagine you have a fasting plan that restricts eating to a specific window each day. What happens if you're invited to a breakfast meeting or a late dinner? This is where you can apply the concept of a flexible fasting window.

If your usual eating window is from noon to 8 pm, but you have a breakfast meeting, consider adjusting your window to start earlier on that day. Perhaps from 8 am to 4 pm. The key here is to maintain the length of your fasting period. This adjustment ensures that you can engage in social events without feeling restricted by your fasting plan.

Travel often disrupts regular schedules. Whether it's a vacation or a business trip, the change in time zones, dining options, and general routine can make sticking to a strict fasting schedule challenging. Prepare for this by planning ahead. If you know you'll be in a different time zone, start adjusting your eating window a few days before your trip to more closely align with your destination's local time. This gradual shift can help your body adapt more smoothly and reduce stress around meal planning when you arrive.

Listening to your body is paramount. There are days when you might feel more hungry or less energetic. On these days, it's beneficial to reassess your fasting plan. If you typically follow a 16/8 fasting schedule and find yourself struggling with energy levels, it might be helpful to shorten your fasting window to 14/10 for a while. Paying attention to your body's signals does not mean you are compromising your goals. Instead, you are ensuring that your approach to fasting is always aligned with what your body needs to stay healthy and vibrant.

Additionally, if you feel unwell or if fasting is making you uncomfortable beyond the usual initial challenges, it's wise to consult with a healthcare provider. They can offer guidance tailored to your specific health needs and circumstances. Remember, the goal of fasting is to improve your health, not to add undue stress or discomfort to your life.

Another aspect of flexibility involves nutritional intake during your eating windows. It's crucial to focus on balanced, nutrient-dense foods that provide your body with the energy and substances it needs to thrive. However, if you find yourself at a social event where the food options don't completely align with these principles, it's okay to make the best choices available and enjoy the moment. A single meal won't derail your progress if the majority of your diet remains aligned with your health objectives.

Consider keeping a fasting journal. This tool can be incredibly helpful for noting down how different adjustments affect your body and mind. If you adjust your eating window for a social occasion, jot down any changes in how you feel or in your energy levels. This practice can provide insightful data over time, helping you to understand which types of flexibility work best for you.

Finally, remember that consistency over time is more important than perfection in any single day. Life is fluid, and your fasting plan should be too. By allowing for adjustments and listening to your body, you reinforce the sustainability of your health journey. This approach not only makes the process more manageable but also more enjoyable. Fasting is not just a regimen; it’s a lifestyle that should enhance your life, not complicate it.

In conclusion, integrating flexibility into your fasting practice is essential for managing the realities of everyday life while still pursuing your health goals. By planning ahead for travel, adjusting your fasting windows to accommodate social situations, listening to your body, and maintaining a balanced diet, you can sustain a fasting regimen that supports your overall wellbeing and longevity. Keep these strategies in mind as you continue to explore and refine your approach to fasting, ensuring it remains a beneficial and adaptable part of your lifestyle.

Setting Goals and Tracking Progress

When you embark on a journey, it is essential to know where you are heading and to track your progress along the way. This is true whether you are traveling, learning a new skill, or improving your health, particularly in managing or preventing cardiovascular diseases through fasting. Setting specific, measurable goals and tracking your progress can significantly enhance your ability to succeed in your fasting endeavors.

Firstly, let's talk about the importance of setting specific and measurable goals for your fasting plan. These goals are not just about how long you can go without eating. Instead, they should focus on the outcomes you want to achieve, such as improving your heart health, losing weight, or lowering your cholesterol levels. By setting clear and precise goals, you give yourself a target to aim for and a clear criterion by which to measure your success.

To set a specific goal, start by defining what you want to accomplish with your fasting plan. Do you want to reduce your blood pressure? Are you looking to decrease inflammatory markers in your blood? Or perhaps your goal is to enhance overall cardiovascular fitness? Once you have identified your goal, make it as specific as possible. For example, rather than saying, "I want to lower my blood pressure," a more specific goal would be, "I want to reduce my systolic blood pressure by 20 points."

After setting specific goals, the next step is to ensure these goals are measurable. This means you should be able to track your progress in a tangible way. Continuing with the blood pressure example, you can measure your progress by regularly checking your blood pressure with a reliable monitor. Keeping a record of each reading will help you see if the changes in your fasting routine are helping you move towards your goal.

Tracking your progress is crucial, not just for motivation but also for evaluating the effectiveness of your fasting plan. This is where a fasting journal comes into play. Keeping a fasting journal allows you to record not only your fasting hours and what you eat during your eating windows but also how you feel physically and mentally. Over time, this journal will provide invaluable insights into how fasting affects your body and mind. It can help you identify patterns or changes that might necessitate adjustments to your fasting schedule or nutrition plan.

In addition to a fasting journal, monitoring health markers related to cardiovascular diseases is highly beneficial. These health markers can include your blood pressure, cholesterol levels, blood sugar levels, and body mass index (BMI). Regular check-ups with your healthcare provider to monitor these markers can inform you about your body's response to your fasting regime and whether you are moving closer to or further from your cardiovascular health goals.

Moreover, tracking these health markers can also provide motivation. Seeing tangible improvements in your health metrics can reinforce the benefits of your fasting plan, encouraging you to continue and even intensify your efforts. For instance, witnessing a significant drop in cholesterol levels after a few months of fasting can be a powerful motivator to maintain or enhance your fasting schedule.

To make this process as effective as possible, consider using digital tools and apps designed for health tracking. Many apps can help you log your food intake, fasting periods, and health markers all in one place. These tools often provide visual representations of your progress, such as graphs and charts, which can make it easier to see trends and make informed decisions about your health regimen.

Finally, remember that the journey to better cardiovascular health through fasting is a personal one. While it's important to set goals and track progress, it's equally important to listen to your body and adjust your plan as needed. Regularly review your fasting journal and health markers, discuss them with your healthcare provider, and make adjustments where necessary. Your body will often tell you what it needs; your job is to listen and adapt accordingly.

By setting specific and measurable goals, keeping a detailed fasting journal, and regularly monitoring health markers, you equip yourself with the tools to make informed decisions about your health. This structured approach will not only help you manage or prevent cardiovascular diseases but also empower you to take control of your health and well-being in a proactive manner.

Chapter Recap

In the chapters we've covered so far, we've explored various aspects of designing your personalized fasting plan. This plan is not just any routine; it's tailored specifically to fit into your life, respecting the demands and uniqueness of your daily activities and responsibilities. Let's take a moment to summarize the key components involved in crafting a fasting schedule that aligns with your lifestyle and dietary needs, ensuring you're set up for success in enhancing your cardiovascular health.

Initially, we assessed your lifestyle, considering how your work schedule, family obligations, and personal routines might affect your ability to maintain a fasting protocol. Recognizing these factors is crucial because a plan that doesn't fit your lifestyle is challenging to maintain. Next, we compared different fasting methods like the 16/8 method and the 5:2 approach. This comparison was vital to help you select a fasting protocol that you can sustain over the long term without feeling overwhelmed or overly restricted.

Following the selection of a fasting method, we planned your meals and nutrition. This step was about ensuring that during your eating windows, your meals are balanced and nutrient-dense. The goal here is not merely to restrict eating times but to nourish your body optimally when you do eat. This approach supports your heart health and overall well-being by making sure that you're not just cutting calories, but you're consuming foods that enrich your body with vitamins, minerals, and other essential nutrients.

Moreover, we discussed the importance of allowing for flexibility in your fasting plan. Life events, travel, and social occasions will happen, and your ability to adapt to these situations without completely falling off the plan is key to your long-term success. Flexibility prevents discouragement and helps in maintaining a healthier lifestyle without feeling like you're sacrificing every social joy life has to offer.

Finally, we talked about setting specific, measurable goals and keeping a track of your progress through a fasting journal. This monitoring is not just about ensuring adherence to the fasting schedule but also about observing how your body responds to the plan. It's about empowering you with knowledge about what works best for your body and adapting based on that feedback.

Now, let's talk about action steps you can take to create a weekly fasting schedule that makes sense for you:

- **Review Your Calendar:** Start by looking at your weekly commitments. Identify days with fewer obligations where beginning a fasting protocol might be easier.
- **Choose Your Protocol:** Based on your lifestyle assessment, select a fasting method that fits best. For instance, if your mornings are busy, an afternoon-to-evening eating window might

work better.

- **Plan Your Meals:** Outline what nutrient-dense meals you will have during your eating windows. It can be helpful to prepare these meals in advance or have a meal plan ready to prevent impulsive eating.
- **Set Clear Goals:** Define what you aim to achieve with your fasting plan. Whether it's weight loss, improved metabolic health, or better heart function, having clear goals will keep you motivated.
- **Track Your Progress:** Keep a journal of your fasting days, how you feel, and any changes in your health parameters. This record-keeping will help you stay on track and make necessary adjustments.
- **Stay Flexible and Adapt:** Be prepared to modify your fasting schedule based on your body's response and any changes in your routine. Flexibility is crucial in making the fasting lifestyle a sustainable practice.

By following these steps, you are not just experimenting with intermittent fasting; you are integrating it into your life in a way that supports your heart health and overall well-being. Remember, the goal of adopting a fasting plan is not to add more stress to your life but to enhance your health and longevity in a manageable and sustainable way. Your fasting plan should feel like a natural part of your life, something that you can maintain without feeling deprived or overwhelmed.

As you move forward, keep in mind that the journey to better health is a marathon, not a sprint. It's about making incremental changes that add up over time, leading to substantial health benefits. With the right plan, a clear understanding of your body's needs, and a commitment to adapt as necessary, you can achieve a healthier heart and a more vibrant life.

Let this chapter serve as a guide to help you craft a fasting approach that resonates with your lifestyle and supports your cardiovascular health. By customizing your fasting schedule, focusing on nutritious food intake, and being adaptable, you're setting yourself up for success in your health journey.

Exercise for Heart Health

The Cardiovascular Benefits of Exercise

Exercise plays a crucial role in maintaining and enhancing heart health. It does so by strengthening the heart and blood vessels, which are vital components of the cardiovascular system. This system is responsible for the circulation of blood throughout the body, and keeping it healthy is essential for overall well-being.

When you engage in physical activity, your heart rate increases. This is your heart working harder to pump blood to muscles and organs that are in action. Over time, this increased demand helps to strengthen the heart muscle itself, similar to how lifting weights improves muscle strength. A strong heart can pump more blood with less effort, which reduces the strain on the heart and helps prevent heart disease.

Besides strengthening the heart, exercise also contributes to better blood vessels. Physical activity promotes the dilation of blood vessels, improving their ability to expand and contract. Healthy blood vessels improve blood flow and reduce the risk of vascular diseases such as atherosclerosis, where arteries become clogged by fatty substances. Moreover, exercise helps in reducing blood pressure, a major risk factor for heart attacks and strokes.

One of the most significant benefits of regular exercise is the improvement it brings in circulation and oxygen delivery to various parts of the body. With better circulation, your cells receive more oxygen and nutrients. This not only boosts the functionality of organs but also aids in the efficient removal of waste products. Enhanced oxygen delivery is particularly important for heart health because it helps the heart muscle function better and reduces the risk of heart disease complications.

Engaging in regular physical activity also has a role in the management of cholesterol levels. It helps increase the levels of high-density lipoprotein (HDL), often referred to as 'good' cholesterol, which helps remove other forms of cholesterol from your bloodstream. Additionally, exercise can lower levels of low-density lipoprotein (LDL), known as 'bad' cholesterol, which can build up in arteries and lead to heart disease.

The benefits of exercise are not instantaneous but accrue over time with consistent practice. Each session of physical activity contributes to this protective effect, making regularity crucial for sustained cardiovascular health. It's important to note that the type and intensity of exercise can influence these benefits, which is why understanding what forms of exercise are most effective for cardiovascular health is key.

By now, you might be wondering how much exercise is enough to reap these cardiovascular benefits. While there is no one-size-fits-all answer, general guidelines suggest that adults should aim for at least 150 minutes of moderate-intensity aerobic exercise, or 75 minutes of vigorous-intensity aerobic exercise each week. Activities could include walking, swimming, cycling, or other forms of dynamic movement that increase heart rate and stimulate cardiovascular functions.

Integrating exercise into your routine can seem challenging, especially if you are starting out or have a busy schedule. However, the key is to find activities that you enjoy and can stick to over the long term. Remember, the goal is to maintain and improve your heart health, so consistency is more important than intensity in the beginning.

In conclusion, the role of exercise in promoting heart health cannot be overstated. By strengthening the heart and improving blood vessel function, exercise helps to enhance blood circulation and oxygen delivery, which are fundamental for maintaining cardiovascular health. Regular physical activity not only helps prevent heart-related diseases but also contributes to a better quality of life by improving overall physical and mental health. Making exercise a regular part of your life is a powerful step towards a healthier heart.

Types of Exercise for Cardiovascular Health

When you think about exercise for cardiovascular health, the two main categories that come to our mind are aerobic activities and resistance training. Each form of exercise provides unique benefits to the heart and overall health, making them essential components in a cardiovascular health regimen.

Aerobic activities, often referred to as cardio, are exercises that increase your heart rate and keep it elevated for a period. These activities primarily help to improve the endurance of your heart muscle. This is crucial because a strong heart pumps blood more efficiently, reducing the strain on your heart and ultimately helping to prevent heart-related issues. Walking, running, cycling, swimming, and dancing fall under this category. Engaging in these activities leads to improved use of oxygen by your muscles, which is great for your heart's health. For adults over 40, the key is to start at a comfortable pace and gradually increase the intensity. This approach helps to build endurance safely while reducing the risk of injuries.

On the other hand, resistance training, which involves activities like weight lifting, using resistance bands, or performing body-weight exercises such as push-ups and squats, focuses more on muscular strength. You might wonder how strengthening your muscles relates to heart health. Strong muscles help you perform daily activities more efficiently, which reduces the burden on your heart. Additionally, resistance training helps improve metabolic health, which is crucial for weight management, reducing the risk of type 2 diabetes, and ultimately, keeping your heart healthy.

Another significant benefit of resistance training is its role in improving your body composition - the ratio of fat to muscle. Lower body fat percentage often correlates with decreased risk for cardiovascular diseases. Resistance training also helps in increasing bone density, which is particularly important as you age and your bones start to weaken.

For someone in their 40s or older, it is advisable to engage in moderate resistance training, focusing on all major muscle groups. This should be done at least two days a week. It is important to stress the need for proper form to prevent injuries. If you are new to resistance training, consider starting with lighter weights or resistance bands, and gradually increase the resistance as your strength improves.

Both aerobic and resistance exercises have their place in a heart-healthy exercise regimen. For optimal benefits, a combination of both is recommended. This ensures not only cardiovascular endurance but also overall strength and metabolic health which are all important for longevity and a good quality of life. As you plan your exercise routine, consider your current fitness level, any existing health conditions, and, ideally, consult with a healthcare provider or a fitness expert to design a program that's safe and effective for you.

Remember, the goal is to make exercise a regular part of your life. This consistency over time is what leads to significant improvements in cardiovascular health and general well-being. Starting slow, setting realistic goals, and progressively challenging yourself as you become fitter will help keep you motivated and reduce the risk of burnout or injury.

In conclusion, understanding and implementing the right types of exercises for your cardiovascular health can lead to profound benefits. Aerobic activities will help improve the efficiency of your heart and lungs, while resistance training will strengthen your muscles and improve metabolic health. Together, they form a comprehensive approach to maintaining and enhancing heart health. By incorporating both types of exercises into your weekly routine, you are not only working towards a healthier heart but also improving your overall health and paving the way for a more active and fulfilling life.

Guidelines and Recommendations

When considering exercise for heart health, understanding how often, how intensely, and for how long you should exercise is crucial. These guidelines provide a structured approach to ensure safety and effectiveness, particularly for adults over 40 who are focused on preventing or managing cardiovascular diseases. This section aims to equip you with practical and actionable advice to incorporate exercise into your routine safely and effectively.

Firstly, let's talk about the frequency of exercise. Ideally, adults should aim to engage in some form of physical activity every day. However, the American Heart Association suggests at least 150 minutes of moderate aerobic exercise per week, or 75 minutes of vigorous exercise. This can be broken down into about 30 minutes a day, five days a week. Consistency is key in maintaining cardiovascular health, so setting a regular schedule helps in creating a routine you can stick to.

Next, the intensity of the exercise should be considered. Moderate intensity means you are moving enough to raise your heart rate and break a sweat. You should still be able to talk but not sing the words to your favorite song. Examples include brisk walking, slow biking, or water aerobics. Vigorous activities, where talking becomes difficult, include jogging, swimming laps, or cycling at a faster pace. It's important to gradually build up intensity to avoid overexertion, especially if you are new to regular exercise or have pre-existing health concerns.

The duration of exercise is also important. While the 30 minutes per day guideline is beneficial, it's worth noting that this can be broken up into shorter segments. Three 10-minute sessions of activity can be just as effective as one 30-minute session. This approach can help manage fatigue and reduce the risk of injury, making it a practical option for those who may find a continuous 30-minute session daunting.

Age-specific considerations must also be taken into account. As you age, your body responds differently to exercise. Those over 40 should ensure they include flexibility and balance exercises, which are crucial for preventing falls and injuries. Also, incorporating strength training at least two days per week helps maintain muscle mass and support metabolic health, which are both important as you age. It's advisable to consult with a healthcare provider before starting any new exercise regimen, especially if you have any chronic health conditions or concerns.

Safety is paramount. Always warm up before exercising to prepare your body and reduce the risk of injury. A simple warm-up could include light walking, slowly moving the limbs, or stretching major muscle groups. Cooling down after exercise with similar light activities helps in the recovery process and ensures a smoother transition back to your daily activities.

Lastly, make adjustments as needed. Listen to your body and adjust the frequency, intensity, and duration of your exercise based on how you feel. It's normal to have varying levels of energy and capability, so being flexible with your routine can help maintain a consistent exercise habit without causing burnout or injury. Regular assessments with health professionals can also help tailor your exercise program to better suit your cardiovascular health needs.

In conclusion, following these guidelines will help you develop an exercise routine that supports heart health while considering your age and individual health status. Remember, the key to benefiting from exercise is consistency, so focus on finding activities that you enjoy and can regularly participate in. This approach not only improves your cardiovascular health but also enhances overall quality of life, helping you stay active and energetic as you age.

Sample Exercises and Workouts

When it comes to improving heart health through exercise, knowing where to start can be the hardest part. It's important to choose activities that not only strengthen the heart but are also enjoyable enough to stick with over time. Let's explore some effective cardiovascular exercises that are suitable for all fitness levels, followed by strength training moves that target major muscle groups.

First and foremost, for anyone over 40 looking to either prevent or manage cardiovascular diseases, walking stands out as one of the most accessible exercises. It doesn't require special equipment and can be done almost anywhere. Starting with a simple 30-minute walk daily can make a significant improvement in your heart health. Over time, you can increase the pace or the duration, depending on how comfortable you feel.

Swimming is another excellent cardiovascular workout that's easy on the joints and effective for the heart. It engages multiple muscle groups simultaneously, which helps to build endurance and strength. Try swimming for 20 to 30 minutes a few times a week. You might start with one lap at a time, gradually increasing the number of laps as your stamina improves.

Cycling, whether outdoor or on a stationary bike, is yet another heart-healthy exercise. It's particularly good for those who might prefer a seated activity due to joint issues or other limitations. Starting with as little as 10 to 15 minutes a day and increasing the duration and intensity as your fitness level allows can greatly benefit your cardiovascular health.

Now, let's talk about strength training, which is equally important for maintaining a healthy heart. Strength training helps not just in building muscle mass but also improving metabolic rate and enhancing the ability of the heart to work efficiently under stress. Incorporating simple bodyweight exercises like squats, push-ups, and lunges can make a big difference. Begin with sets of 10 for each exercise, slowly building up the number of sets and repetitions over weeks and months.

For those who might be more experienced or looking for variety, incorporating resistance bands or light dumbbells can add additional resistance and help improve muscular strength and endurance further. Exercises like bicep curls, tricep extensions, and light dumbbell presses are great. It is crucial to focus on form to prevent any injuries. You can start with two sets of 10 to 12 repetitions for each of these exercises, gradually increasing as you become more comfortable.

It's also beneficial to include some flexibility and balance exercises in your routine. Yoga and tai chi are excellent for enhancing flexibility, reducing stress, and improving cardiovascular health. They also help in maintaining muscle tone and promoting blood flow. Starting with basic poses and forms, and joining a class or following a video at home can make these exercises more enjoyable and effective.

Finally, it's essential to remember that consistency is key. Integrating these exercises into your weekly routine, and gradually increasing the intensity and frequency, will contribute significantly to your cardiovascular health. Always consult with your healthcare provider before starting any new exercise regimen, especially if you have pre-existing health conditions or concerns.

By incorporating a mix of cardiovascular and strength training exercises, you can create a balanced workout routine that not only boosts your heart health but also improves overall physical fitness and wellbeing. Remember, the goal is to find activities that you enjoy and can stick with long term. This will not only help in managing or preventing cardiovascular diseases but also enhance your quality of life as you age.

Progression and Consistency

When it comes to improving heart health through exercise, progression and consistency are two foundational principles that can greatly enhance the effectiveness of your fitness routine. Understanding these concepts is critical for anyone looking to prevent or manage cardiovascular diseases.

Progression in exercise means gradually increasing the intensity, duration, and complexity of your workouts over time. This principle is based on the body's natural ability to adapt to stress. By slowly increasing the demands placed on your heart and muscles, you encourage adaptations such as increased cardiovascular efficiency and stronger muscles.

Let’s talk about why this gradual increase is important. If you start with too much intensity or for too long, you risk injury or excessive fatigue, which can discourage you from continuing. It’s like trying to lift a weight that’s far too heavy; trying to do too much too soon can lead to setbacks rather than progress.

To implement progression, you might start with walking for 10-15 minutes a day. After doing this consistently for a week or two, you could increase to 20 minutes a day, or begin including short intervals of brisk walking. Each week or two, assess how you feel and adjust accordingly. The key is small increases. These small steps lead to big changes without overwhelming your body or your schedule.

Consistency, on the other hand, refers to the frequency of your exercises. Exercising consistently helps establish a routine, making it more likely that you will stick with your exercise program long-term. More importantly, regular physical activity is essential to maintain the physiological benefits gained from exercise.

Why is this regularity so crucial? Imagine your body as a machine that runs smoother with regular use. Without consistent exercise, the benefits such as improved blood circulation and increased heart strength begin to decrease. Think of it as a 'use it or lose it' scenario where consistency keeps the engine running smoothly.

To cultivate consistency, it’s helpful to schedule your exercise times just as you would any other important appointment. This might mean setting aside specific times of the day or days of the week for physical activity. It’s also beneficial to incorporate a variety of exercises that you enjoy, which can make the routine less monotonous and more enjoyable.

Another tip is to set achievable goals. These goals can be daily, weekly, or monthly. For example, you might aim to walk a certain number of steps each day or to attend three fitness classes per week. Tracking your progress towards these goals can provide motivation and a sense of accomplishment that encourages further consistency.

The combination of progression and consistency in an exercise regimen creates a powerful tool for improving cardiovascular health. As you gradually increase your exercise intensity and remain consistent with your routines, your body adapts. These adaptations include stronger heart muscles and improved circulation, which significantly reduce the risk of heart diseases.

Moreover, the psychological benefits of exercise, such as reduced stress and improved mood, also contribute to cardiovascular health. Consistent exercise helps manage stress hormones like cortisol, which when left unchecked, can contribute to heart issues.

In conclusion, remember that starting slow and building up gradually while sticking to a regular schedule will make your journey towards a healthier heart more effective and enjoyable. By understanding and applying the principles of progression and consistency, you can enhance your heart health, boost your overall wellbeing, and enjoy a more active lifestyle well into your later years.

To get started, choose activities you enjoy and start small. Keep track of your progress and adjust as you become fitter. Most importantly, try to stay consistent, even when it feels challenging. Over time, these steps will become a natural part of your lifestyle, leading to a healthier heart and a better quality of life.

Chapter Recap

Throughout this chapter, we have explored the significant impact that exercise has on maintaining and improving cardiovascular health. Let's take a moment to recap the key principles we've covered regarding exercise and its benefits for your heart. Understanding these will help you in making informed decisions about integrating physical activity into your daily life.

Exercise serves as a powerful tool in strengthening the heart and the entire circulatory system. Regular physical activity helps in enhancing the heart's efficiency - it pumps more blood per beat. Improved circulation means that your body gets better at delivering oxygen and nutrients to various tissues, and at the same time, it becomes more proficient at removing waste products. This enhanced efficiency contributes significantly to your overall health and wellbeing.

We discussed different types of exercises that benefit cardiovascular health. Aerobic exercises like walking, cycling, swimming, and jogging are particularly effective in improving the endurance of your heart. These activities keep your heart rate elevated for extended periods, which is excellent for building a strong cardiovascular system. On the other hand, resistance training, which includes activities like lifting weights or using resistance bands, helps in maintaining muscular strength and metabolic health. These exercises are essential as they support the structure and function of your blood vessels.

It's important to follow certain guidelines to get the most out of your exercise routines safely. We talked about the ideal frequency, intensity, and duration of exercise sessions. Ideally, adults should engage in at least 150 minutes of moderate-intensity aerobic physical activity throughout the week, or at least 75 minutes of vigorous-intensity aerobic physical activity, or an equivalent combination of both. Adding muscle-strengthening activities on two or more days a week enhances the benefits. We also considered age-specific considerations to ensure that your training is safe and appropriate for your fitness level.

Now, let us move to some practical advice. To make these principles work for you, here are some actionable steps you can start implementing right away:

- Schedule your exercise sessions in your calendar as you would any important appointment. This makes it more likely that you will stick to your plan.
- Start with moderate exercises if you are not used to regular physical activity. Gradually increase the intensity and duration as your body adapts.
- Include a variety of exercises. Mix aerobic activities with resistance training to balance the benefits across your heart, lungs, and muscles.
- Stay consistent. Try to exercise at the same time each day to establish a routine that becomes a regular part of your life.

- Keep track of your progress. Note your exercise durations, the intensity of your workouts, and how you feel after each session. This will help you adjust your activities to better suit your needs and goals.

Exercise is a cornerstone of good cardiovascular health. By integrating regular physical activity into your routine, you actively contribute to the longevity and quality of your life. Remember, each step you take is a step towards a healthier heart. Start slow, be consistent, and gradually build up your strength and endurance. Your heart, the vital organ that keeps you going, will thank you for your perseverance and care.

As we conclude this chapter, keep in mind that the journey to better heart health through exercise is a marathon, not a sprint. It's about making gradual, consistent changes to your lifestyle that add up to substantial benefits over time. Make exercise a non-negotiable part of your life, just like eating and sleeping. With these steps in mind, you're not just exercising, you're cultivating a heart-healthy lifestyle.

Creating Your Exercise Plan

Evaluating Your Current Fitness Level

Before embarking on any new exercise routine, it's crucial to understand where you currently stand in terms of fitness. This initial step isn't just about setting a baseline but ensuring that the exercise plan you adopt is both safe and effective for your specific health circumstances, particularly if you are over 40 and concerned about cardiovascular health.

To begin evaluating your fitness level, focus first on your cardiovascular endurance. This is the ability of your heart and lungs to work together to fuel your body with oxygen during prolonged physical activity. Understanding your current cardiovascular endurance can help determine how much you can handle when you start exercising. A simple way to assess this is by seeing how long you can briskly walk or jog without stopping. The time you manage to sustain this activity gives a rough estimate of your cardiovascular health.

Another aspect of evaluating your current fitness is strength assessment. Testing your strength can be as straightforward as checking how many standard push-ups or sit-ups you can perform in a row. The number of repetitions you complete provides insight into your muscle strength and endurance. These exercises target multiple muscle groups and offer a snapshot of your overall physical strength.

It's also vital to identify any limitations or health concerns before starting an exercise plan. This means taking into account any current or past injuries, chronic health issues such as heart conditions or arthritis, or any recommendations from your healthcare provider. Knowing these can help tailor your exercise plan to avoid aggravating existing conditions and focus on improving your health safely.

For instance, if you have been diagnosed with high blood pressure, certain exercises like heavy weight lifting might be initially off-limits. Instead, you could focus on lower-impact cardiovascular exercises such as walking or swimming, which are less stressful on your cardiovascular system but effective in building endurance.

By starting with a thorough evaluation of your cardiovascular endurance, strength, and any physical limitations, you are setting a foundation for a personalized and effective exercise plan. This approach not only helps in preventing injuries but also ensures that you progress towards better cardiovascular health at a pace that is right for you.

Moreover, understanding your starting point allows you to measure progress as you get into your exercise routine. It's not just about reaching a destination but also appreciating the journey of getting fitter and healthier. Each small improvement is a step towards enhancing your quality of life and managing or preventing cardiovascular diseases.

So, take the time to assess your fitness level accurately. It's an essential first step that directs you to a path of successful and healthy physical activity. Remember, the goal is to improve your longevity and quality of life through manageable and enjoyable exercise routines that are tailored specifically to your health needs and fitness level.

Setting Realistic Fitness Goals

When it comes to improving cardiovascular health and overall quality of life, setting realistic fitness goals is a crucial step. To begin with, it's important to understand what realistic fitness goals look like and why they matter. A realistic fitness goal is one that you can achieve within your current physical and time limitations, considering your overall health condition. For someone over 40, this could mean starting with goals that are moderate and gradually increasing the intensity and duration of exercise based on how your body responds.

Short-term goals are your stepping stones. They are the immediate, smaller achievements that pave the way to your long-term aspirations. For example, a short-term goal might be to walk for 15 minutes a day, five days a week. This is manageable for most people and sets a foundation for increasing activity. It's also essential to align these short-term goals with your fasting plan and lifestyle. If you are practicing intermittent fasting, you might schedule your walks during your eating windows when you have more energy.

Long-term goals focus on the bigger picture. These might include reducing your blood pressure or cholesterol levels, or perhaps being able to complete a 5K run. Long-term goals provide a direction and end point to strive towards, but they are achieved gradually through the accumulation of short-term successes.

Aligning your goals with your fasting plan and lifestyle is about making your health regimen sustainable. If your lifestyle includes busy days with limited time for the gym, your exercise plan needs to reflect that. Perhaps exercising at home or shorter, more intense workouts could work better for you. Aligning your exercise goals with intermittent fasting involves understanding how your body reacts to exercise during fasting periods and what times of day you feel most energetic. This alignment helps in creating a plan that feels less like a schedule and more like a natural part of your day.

Once you set these goals, it's also beneficial to write them down and place them somewhere you can see daily. This acts as a constant reminder of what you're working toward. Also, sharing these goals with a friend or family member can help keep you accountable. They can check in with you on your progress, and you can celebrate small victories together. This support system is invaluable.

It is also wise to reevaluate your goals periodically. This doesn't mean you are lowering your standards if you find certain goals too challenging, but rather ensuring that your goals remain realistic as your fitness level changes, or as other life circumstances evolve. Perhaps you find that you are achieving your initial short-term goals quite easily, and feel ready to increase your exercise time to 30 minutes a day. This adjustment is both a sign of your progress and an opportunity to push your limits a bit further, safely and effectively.

Finally, remember that setbacks are normal, and adjusting your goals isn't a sign of failure but rather a part of the journey to better health. If you experience a health issue or find that your initial goals were too ambitious, it's perfectly okay to scale back. The key is to keep moving forward, even if it's at a slower pace than originally planned. This approach not only keeps you physically active but also boosts your morale by allowing you to meet the targets you set, fostering a sense of achievement and encouraging persistence.

In conclusion, setting realistic fitness goals as an adult over 40 is about understanding your body, aligning your exercise with your lifestyle, and being flexible enough to adjust as needed. These goals not only pave the way to improved physical health but also enhance your overall quality of life, making each day healthier and happier. Keep your goals clear, attainable, and aligned with your lifestyle, and you'll find that maintaining an exercise regimen becomes a more enjoyable and integrated part of your daily routine.

Designing a Balanced Routine

When we talk about creating an exercise routine, the key is to ensure it is balanced. This means that the routine should include different types of exercises. These exercises should help improve both your heart health and muscle strength. It is also important to plan days for rest and recovery. Let's dive into how to create this balanced routine, step by step.

The first step in designing a balanced exercise routine is to understand the different types of exercises. There are mainly two types: aerobic and strength training. Aerobic exercises, such as walking, running, cycling, or swimming, are designed to increase your heart rate. They improve the health of your heart and lungs. Strength exercises, like lifting weights or using resistance bands, focus on building muscle mass and strength.

Why is it important to include both types of exercise? Aerobic exercise helps to reduce your risk of heart disease by lowering blood pressure and cholesterol levels. It also helps in managing weight, which is a major factor in heart health. On the other hand, strength training is equally important. It helps you maintain muscle mass, which naturally declines as you age. Strong muscles are not just about looking good. They are also crucial for performing everyday activities easily and safely.

Now, let's talk about planning your routine. It is beneficial to mix these exercises throughout the week. For example, you might decide to do aerobic exercises on Monday, Wednesday, and Friday. Then, you could set Tuesday and Thursday for strength training. This schedule gives your body the chance to engage in both types of exercises without overstraining any specific muscle group.

Incorporating rest days is as important as planning workout days. Why? Because when you exercise, especially during strength training, your muscle fibers get small tears. These tears are normal, but they need time to heal. This healing process helps the muscles to become stronger. Rest days allow this healing to happen. Without them, you risk injuries and fatigue, which can demotivate you and derail your fitness goals.

It is also essential to consider your current fitness level and any health issues you might have. For instance, if you have been inactive for a while, you might want to start with lighter and shorter exercise sessions. Gradually increase the intensity and duration as your fitness improves. If you have any chronic conditions like arthritis or heart disease, consult your doctor before starting any new exercise routine. They can provide guidance on what exercises are safe and beneficial for you.

A balanced routine isn't just about the types of exercises and rest days. It's also about making it part of your daily life. Here are some tips to make it easier to stick to your routine. First, set specific times for your workouts. Treat them as important appointments that you cannot miss. This helps in building a habit. Secondly, mix up your exercises. Doing the same routine can become boring over time. Try different activities to keep your interest alive. Finally, track your progress. This could be noting down the weights you lift, the distance you run, or how you feel after exercising. Seeing improvements can be a huge motivator.

To summarize, a balanced exercise routine is crucial for maintaining cardiovascular health and overall well-being. It should include a mix of aerobic and strength training exercises. Don't forget to schedule rest days to allow your body to recover. Start slow, especially if you are new to exercising, and gradually build up your routine. Remember, the goal is to make exercise a regular and enjoyable part of your life.

By following these steps, you are not just working towards better physical health; you are setting the foundation for a healthier, more active future. Remember, every bit of movement counts. Start where you are, use what you have, and do what you can. Over time, your heart will thank you, and you will feel the rewards of a balanced routine in every step you take.

Warming Up and Cooling Down

When we talk about exercise, warming up and cooling down are two essential components that often get overlooked. Yet, they play a significant role in your overall fitness regimen, especially as we age and our bodies demand more care. Let's delve deep into why these routines matter, and how you can effectively implement them into your exercise plan.

Starting with a warm-up, let's understand what it is and why it is important. A warm-up is a series of activities that gradually increases your heart rate and circulation. This gentle increase helps to loosen the joints and increase blood flow to the muscles that you will be using during your exercise session. By warming up, you are essentially preparing your body for physical activity and reducing your risk of injury. It’s a vital step that helps make the transition into vigorous activities smoother and safer.

Think of your muscles as elastic bands. If an elastic band is cold and you try to quickly stretch it to its limit, it might snap. However, if you gently stretch it gradually, it becomes more pliable and can extend much further without damage. That's exactly what a warm-up does to your muscles.

Now, let’s talk about how to warm up effectively. A good warm-up should last about 5 to 10 minutes and start with very low-intensity movements. For those in our age group, particularly those managing cardiovascular health, starting slow is key. You might begin with walking at a gentle pace or doing a slow march on the spot. Gradually, you can increase the intensity by incorporating more dynamic movements such as leg swings, arm circles, or gentle twists. Remember, the goal is to increase your heart rate slowly and prepare your muscles for the exercises to come, not to tire yourself out before you even start your workout.

After your workout, cooling down is just as crucial as warming up. Cooling down allows your body to gradually return to its normal physiological state. It helps in the recovery process by reducing the buildup of lactic acid, which can lead to muscle stiffness and soreness. Just as you wouldn’t slam on the brakes when driving a car at high speed, you shouldn’t abruptly stop exercising and sit down right away.

A cooling down routine might include walking at a slow pace until your heart rate starts to return to normal. Following this, you can include stretching exercises, which are essential for flexibility and can help reduce muscle tension. Stretching during the cool down also helps to relax the muscles that were intensely used during exercise. Each stretch should be held for about 15 to 30 seconds and should never cause pain. Focus on breathing deeply during your stretches, which helps in reducing heart rate and calming your body.

Here are some specific stretches you can do during your cool down: you might consider a calf stretch, which involves placing one leg behind you with the toe pointed slightly inward and the heel down, then leaning into the wall until you feel a stretch in the back leg's calf. Another good stretch is the hamstring stretch, which can be performed by sitting on the ground and reaching towards your toes, or by placing your foot on a low step and leaning forward gently.

Understanding the importance of warming up and cooling down is fundamental to any exercise routine. These practices not only make your workouts more effective but also safeguard your body against injuries, and, importantly, they are crucial for your cardiovascular health. By incorporating thoughtful, gentle beginnings and endings into your exercise regimen, you're not only looking after your immediate workout effectiveness but also your long-term health and mobility.

To wrap it up, always remember that your body is your most valuable asset, especially as you navigate through later decades. Taking care of it with proper warm-ups and cool-downs is not just a recommendation. It's essential. This careful attention to your body before and after a workout will pay off in fewer injuries, less muscle pain, and a more enjoyable, sustainable exercise habit. It's a simple yet profound way to honor your body's needs and contribute actively to your cardiovascular health.

Start each exercise session with a gentle warm-up, transition into your planned activity, and then gradually taper off with a cool down. This rhythmic flow from start to finish not only enhances your physical fitness but also harmonizes with your cardiovascular goals. Remember, each step, from the gentle beginning of a warm-up to the tranquil descent of cooling down, forms an integral part of your journey towards a healthier heart and a more vigorous life.

Staying Motivated and Accountable

One of the most significant factors in ensuring the success of any new habit, including exercise, is staying motivated and holding oneself accountable. When individuals begin an exercise plan, especially adults over the age of 40 looking to prevent or manage cardiovascular diseases, maintaining a steady level of motivation can be the key to prolonged success. Let us delve into practical ways to keep motivated and how to effectively track progress, alongside celebrating milestones.

To start, the concept of tracking progress is foundational. Tracking allows you to see tangible evidence of your efforts, be it through improved endurance, increased strength, or even weight loss. A straightforward way to track progress is by maintaining an exercise log.

This log should include details about what exercises were performed, the duration of the exercise, and the intensity. As the weeks go by, this log will serve as a historical record of your activity and provide motivational boosts as you see your improvements on paper.

Another significant aspect of the exercise log is its role in accountability. By regularly updating this log, you are making a commitment to yourself. It acts as a physical reminder of your exercise goals and the steps you are taking to achieve them. Seeing empty days can serve as a prompt to get moving, and consistently filled pages can fuel your motivation to keep going.

Celebrating milestones is equally essential. Set achievable targets such as walking a certain distance, attending a set number of gym sessions, or reaching a specific weight. Each time you meet a milestone, allow yourself a moment of celebration. This could be anything from treating yourself to a new book, enjoying a special meal, or simply taking a moment to acknowledge your achievement. These celebrations not only serve as rewards but reinforce the positive behavior of regular physical activity.

Finding an exercise buddy or joining a support group can dramatically increase your motivation and accountability. An exercise buddy is someone who shares similar fitness goals with you. This person can be a friend, family member, or even a neighbor. Exercise sessions can become social events, making them more enjoyable and something to look forward to. Moreover, having someone to share your struggles and successes with makes the journey less daunting.

Online forums and local community groups are excellent for finding support and encouragement. Many communities offer walking clubs, yoga classes, or cycling groups that welcome members of all fitness levels. Participating in these groups provides a sense of community and belonging, which can be incredibly motivating. Additionally, these groups often share tips and experiences that can be invaluable in your fitness journey.

In the context of managing or preventing cardiovascular disease, the stakes are undeniably high. The motivation to maintain an active lifestyle should ideally come from the desire to live a healthy, fulfilling life. Understanding the direct impact of exercise on cardiovascular health, such as improved blood circulation, reduced blood pressure, and better cholesterol levels, can serve as a powerful motivator.

Lastly, remember to set realistic expectations. Progress in physical fitness, especially after the age of 40, can be gradual. Celebrating small victories and staying patient with yourself are crucial. Avoid comparing your journey to others, as each individual's body responds differently to exercise. What matters is your commitment to improving your health at your own pace. Your exercise plan is not just a pathway to better physical health but also to greater happiness and satisfaction in life.

By implementing these practical steps, tracking your progress, celebrating milestones, finding a buddy or support group, and setting realistic expectations, you can ensure that your motivation and accountability remain high. These elements are fundamental not just to achieving your fitness goals but to sustaining them long-term, thereby significantly improving your cardiovascular health and overall quality of life.

Chapter Recap

As we conclude this chapter on creating your exercise plan, it's essential to summarize the key points that will help you embark on a journey towards better cardiovascular health and improved quality of life. Remember, each element we've discussed aims to build a routine that not only fits your current lifestyle but also motivates you towards maintaining long-term health.

First, we assessed your current fitness level. This step is crucial because it provides a baseline from which you can measure progress. Knowing your starting point helps in setting achievable and realistic goals, which keeps you motivated. Whether you're a beginner or you have some experience in exercising, understanding your cardiovascular endurance and strength levels is the first step in crafting an exercise plan that works for you.

Next, we moved on to setting realistic fitness goals. Here, the focus was on establishing short-term and long-term objectives that align with your overall health aspirations. These goals are not just about reaching a certain weight or being able to run a particular distance, but they should also aim to integrate smoothly with your fasting plan and lifestyle choices, ensuring a holistic approach to health.

Designing a balanced routine was another critical element. This involves selecting a variety of aerobic and strength exercises to ensure that all muscle groups are worked, and the heart is trained efficiently. Balancing different types of exercises helps prevent boredom, reduces the risk of injury, and enhances overall body strength and stamina. Furthermore, scheduling rest and recovery days is just as important as the workout days themselves to allow your body to heal and grow stronger.

Warming up and cooling down were also discussed. Proper warm-up routines prepare your body for the stresses of exercise, reducing the risk of injury. Cooling down, on the other hand, helps in gradual recovery and normalizing heart rates, which is vital for your cardiovascular health. Including dynamic stretches and gentle post-workout techniques helps achieve these goals effectively.

Lastly, staying motivated and accountable is essential in any fitness journey. We explored how tracking progress and celebrating milestones can keep you motivated. Additionally, having an exercise buddy or a support system can play a significant role in maintaining your exercise routine. This social support not only makes the process enjoyable but also keeps you accountable.

Now, to make all this actionable, here are clear and specific steps to start your new exercise routine:

- Review your current fitness level: Take notes on what exercises you can do comfortably and areas where you feel limited.
- Set your fitness goals: Write down at least two short-term goals (to be achieved in the next 1-3 months) and one long-term goal (to be achieved in the next 6-12 months).
- Create your workout schedule: Plan your weekly routine, including different types of exercises you enjoy, and ensure you have at least one rest day per week.
- Include warm-up and cool-down: For each workout session, allocate at least 10 minutes for warming up and another 10 minutes for cooling down.
- Find a workout partner: Reach out to friends or family members who might be interested in joining you on your fitness journey, or join a local or online fitness community.
- Track your progress: Use a journal or an app to record your workouts and any milestones you reach. This will help you see how far you've come and what needs to be adjusted.
- Celebrate your achievements: Set up a reward system for yourself for reaching your goals. It could be as simple as treating yourself to a movie or getting new workout gear.

By following these steps, you'll not only create a solid foundation for your exercise plan but also enjoy the journey towards a healthier heart and a better life. Remember, the goal is to make exercise a regular, enjoyable part of your day. So, take it one step at a time, and gradually, you will see the transformations not just physically, but mentally and emotionally too.

This chapter has equipped you with the necessary tools to design an exercise routine that is tailored to your needs and goals. As you implement these strategies, keep in mind that consistency is key. It's not about making massive changes overnight but about making small, manageable adjustments that lead to lasting habits. Here's to a healthier heart and a happier you!

Understanding the Role of Diet in Heart Health

The connection between what we eat and the health of our heart is profound and critical. Every morsel of food you consume goes beyond just satisfying hunger. It plays a significant role in determining how well your heart functions. This is especially true for adults over 40, where the risk of cardiovascular diseases starts to rise. Heart health is influenced by various factors, but diet is one element you can control to help manage or even prevent heart-related issues.

Why is diet so crucial for heart health? Your heart is dependent on certain nutrients to function optimally. These nutrients help in managing blood pressure, reducing cholesterol levels, and keeping your arteries clear of blockages. Understanding which nutrients benefit your heart and how they work gives you the power to make informed decisions about what you eat.

Let's delve into the key nutrients that are essential for maintaining a healthy heart. First, there are unsaturated fats. Unlike saturated fats, which can clog your arteries, unsaturated fats can actually help reduce inflammation and cholesterol levels. Foods rich in unsaturated fats include olive oil, avocados, and nuts. Incorporating these into your diet can contribute to a healthier heart.

Another group of heart-healthy nutrients includes fiber. Fiber is not just beneficial for digestion; it also plays a role in controlling cholesterol levels. Soluble fiber, found in oats, beans, and flaxseeds, helps to slow down the absorption of cholesterol in your bloodstream. Making sure your diet includes a good amount of high-fiber foods can greatly benefit your heart.

Antioxidants also play a role in heart health. These substances, which are abundant in fruits and vegetables, can protect your blood vessels from damage and reduce the risk of heart disease. By incorporating a variety of colorful fruits and vegetables into your diet, you're not just adding flavor to your meals, but also providing your heart with the protection it needs.

Moreover, omega-3 fatty acids are renowned for their role in heart health. Found in fatty fish like salmon and mackerel, as well as in flaxseeds and walnuts, omega-3s help reduce triglycerides in the blood, lower blood pressure, and can even decrease the risk of arrhythmias (abnormal heartbeats). Regularly eating foods rich in omega-3 fatty acids can be a game-changer for your heart health.

While understanding what to eat is crucial, knowing what to avoid is equally important. High intake of salt, sugar, and unhealthy fats (mostly found in processed foods) can lead to high blood pressure, high cholesterol, and heart blockages. Therefore, it's essential to not only focus on adding the right foods to your diet but also limiting those that can harm your heart.

Managing your diet for heart health doesn't have to be about strict limitations. Rather, it's about making smarter choices more consistently. This means opting for whole grains over refined ones, choosing lean proteins instead of fatty cuts of meat, and increasing your intake of fruits and vegetables. Remember, small changes in your diet can lead to big benefits for your heart.

The takeaway here is simple yet powerful: by making informed and mindful choices about what you eat, you can significantly reduce your risk of heart disease and improve your overall cardiovascular health. This isn't just about living longer; it's about living better. With a heart-healthy diet, you can enjoy more vitality and energy to do the things you love with the people you cherish.

To start, consider your next meal. Could you replace a processed food item with a heart-healthy alternative? Perhaps swap a snack for a piece of fruit or choose a salad dressed with olive oil instead of a creamy dressing. Every little choice adds up, and it all begins with understanding the role of diet in heart health.

In conclusion, taking control of your diet is a powerful step towards a healthier heart. This section aimed to equip you with the knowledge of why certain foods impact heart health positively or negatively. As you move forward, use this knowledge to make choices that benefit your heart. Your diet is your strongest ally in the fight against heart disease, and by opting for nutritious foods, you're setting the stage for a healthier, more vibrant life.

Embracing a Heart-Healthy Eating Pattern

One of the simplest yet most effective ways to support your heart health is by adopting an eating pattern that focuses on whole, minimally processed foods. This approach involves choosing foods that are as close to their natural state as possible. It means less packaged items and more fresh produce. Why is this important for your heart? Whole foods are packed with nutrients that play a crucial role in maintaining heart function and overall health.

Let's start by discussing what whole foods are. These are foods that have not been heavily processed or altered from their original form. Think of fruits, vegetables, whole grains, nuts, and seeds. These foods are rich in essential nutrients such as fiber, vitamins, minerals, and antioxidants. Each of these nutrients has a specific role in cardiovascular health. For example, fiber helps reduce blood cholesterol levels, a crucial factor in preventing heart disease.

Minimally processed foods are those that have been processed to increase durability and make them easier to use but retain most of their nutritional value. Examples include frozen fruits and vegetables, canned beans without added salt, and dried herbs. Choosing these over highly processed foods, which often contain high levels of sugars, unhealthy fats, and salt, can significantly benefit your heart health.

Incorporating a variety of colorful fruits and vegetables into your diet is another key aspect of a heart-healthy eating pattern. This isn't just to make your plate more appealing. Different colors often represent different types of nutrients that these foods offer. For instance, red fruits and vegetables like tomatoes and red peppers are high in lycopene, an antioxidant that has been linked to reduced rates of certain types of heart disease.

Green vegetables, like spinach and kale, are loaded with lutein, fiber, and other vitamins, which can help maintain arterial flexibility and lower cholesterol. Blue and purple foods, like blueberries and eggplants, contain anthocyanins that can help lower blood pressure and reduce the risk of heart disease. By eating a rainbow of foods, you ensure a broad intake of these and many other heart-protective nutrients.

Apart from colors, it's crucial to think about the balance of the food you eat. A heart-healthy diet isn't just about adding more fruits and vegetables but also about reducing intake of unhealthy foods. Minimizing the consumption of red meat, processed meats, and high-fat dairy products can reduce the risk of heart issues. Instead, opt for leaner proteins like fish, chicken, and legumes, which provide essential nutrients without excessive saturated fat.

Another essential feature of heart-healthy eating is the type of fats consumed. Not all fats are bad for you. In fact, monounsaturated and polyunsaturated fats, which are found in olive oil, avocados, and nuts, can help reduce bad cholesterol levels and lower the risk of heart disease. However, trans fats found in many baked goods and fried foods should be avoided as they can increase heart disease risk.

Consider also the role of whole grains. Swapping out refined grains like white bread and rice with whole grains such as quinoa, brown rice, and whole wheat can help maintain healthy blood pressure and heart function. Whole grains are a good source of fiber, which again, plays a significant role in managing cholesterol levels.

Lastly, hydration is vital. While not often directly connected to heart health, staying well-hydrated helps your heart pump blood more easily throughout your body and helps muscles work efficiently. This could be as simple as replacing sugary beverages with water or herbal teas that contribute to your overall fluid intake without adding calories or harmful sugars.

By focusing on whole, minimally processed foods and incorporating a variety of colorful fruits and vegetables, you are taking significant steps toward a heart-healthy eating pattern. Each small change you make builds up over time, contributing to better heart health and a higher quality of life. Remember, each meal is an opportunity to benefit your heart. Choose wisely and enjoy the variety of tastes and textures that come with eating for your heart's health.

Adopting these eating patterns does not mean overhauling your entire diet overnight. Start small. Perhaps introduce one new vegetable or fruit into your diet each week. Experiment with replacing processed snack foods with nuts or seeds. Gradually, these small changes will form new habits, making heart-healthy eating a natural part of your life. This is not just about avoiding disease; it's about thriving, feeling good, and enjoying your life with each nutritious meal you consume.

Managing Portion Sizes and Calorie Intake

When we talk about maintaining a healthy heart, managing portion sizes and balancing calorie intake becomes vital. It's not just about what you eat, but also how much you eat that can impact your cardiovascular health. This concept may seem straightforward, but it involves a deeper understanding of your body's needs and the energy provided by food.

Let's start with portion control, which is simply how much food you choose to eat at one time. Overeating is a common issue, often because the body's cues for fullness can be slow to catch up with the rapid pace at which we can consume food. This delay can lead to consuming more calories than we need, which the body then stores as fat. Excess body fat, especially around the abdomen, increases the risk of developing heart disease and other health complications.

Visual cues can serve as practical tools to manage portion sizes without feeling deprived. For instance, a portion of meat should be about the size of a deck of cards, and a serving of vegetables should be about the size of your fist. These comparisons are easy to remember and can help you when you're serving your meals at home.

Mindful eating is another important strategy. It involves paying full attention to the experience of eating and drinking. You focus on the smell, taste, and texture of your food, and you become more aware of how your stomach feels as it fills. This practice can help you recognize when you are full, reducing the likelihood of overeating.

Now, let's discuss calorie intake. Calories are a measure of energy, and balancing the energy you consume with the energy you expend is crucial for maintaining a healthy weight. Consuming more calories than you burn can lead to weight gain, whereas consuming fewer calories than you burn can lead to weight loss.

To manage your calorie intake, first understand how many calories your body needs each day. This varies depending on age, sex, weight, height, and physical activity level. Generally, men need more calories than women, younger adults need more calories than older adults, and those who are more active need more calories than those who are sedentary.

Balancing your calorie intake with physical activity is a dynamic way to manage your weight and support heart health. Any physical activity, from walking to more vigorous exercises, helps burn calories. The key is consistency and enjoyment, which help in maintaining an active lifestyle long term.

Here are some specific, actionable steps you can take to effectively manage portion sizes and calorie intake:

1. Use smaller plates for your meals. Smaller plates can help make smaller portions look larger, and if your plate looks full, you might feel more satisfied even if you're eating less.

2. Read nutrition labels when shopping. Pay attention to the

serving size and the number of servings in the package. Nutrition labels can help you understand how many calories and how much fat, cholesterol, sodium, and other ingredients are in one serving of food.

3. Prepare meals at home. You can control the ingredients and the portion size. Preparing meals at home also helps you make healthier choices and saves you money.

4. When eating out, you can ask for half of your meal to be boxed up before you start eating, or share a meal with someone. This can help manage portion sizes.

5. Increase your physical activity. It can help you balance your calorie intake and use up stored fat as energy. This is important for weight management and heart health.

By understanding and implementing these strategies in your daily life, you can maintain a healthier weight, reduce your risk of heart disease, and improve your overall quality of life. Remember, every small change you make contributes to a bigger impact on your long-term health.

Making Smart Choices When Dining Out

Making smart choices when dining out is crucial, especially for those of us over 40 looking to manage or prevent cardiovascular diseases. Eating out can pose a challenge because it often involves high-calorie meals that are rich in unhealthy fats, salts, and sugars. However, with the right strategies, you can enjoy dining out without compromising your heart health.

Firstly, navigating restaurant menus smartly is essential. When you look at a menu, try to identify dishes that are cooked in healthier ways. For example, options that are grilled, steamed, or baked are typically healthier than foods that are fried or sautéed. Restaurants often use a lot of butter and oil in sautéed dishes, which can add unnecessary fats to your meal.

Choosing dishes that emphasize vegetables can also make a big difference. Vegetables are low in calories and high in dietary fiber, vitamins, and minerals that support heart health. Look for dishes where vegetables are the main component, not just a side dish. This can include options like salads, vegetable stir-fries, or dishes where vegetables are mixed with whole grains like quinoa or brown rice.

When it comes to making heart-healthy substitutions, don't hesitate to ask for changes to your meal. Most restaurants are willing to accommodate simple requests such as dressing on the side or substituting a side of fries with a salad or extra vegetables. This can significantly reduce the calorie content of your meal while increasing its nutritional value.

Another important aspect of dining out is portion control. Restaurant portions can be quite large, and it's easy to eat more than intended. One way to manage portion sizes is to ask for a half portion or a children's size if available. Alternatively, you could share a dish with someone else at your table or ask for a box at the beginning of the meal and pack away half to take home for another meal.

Practicing moderation is vital, especially in social settings where there might be multiple courses or a variety of dishes on offer. It's okay to enjoy a small portion of something indulgent, but balance it out with healthier choices throughout the rest of the meal. For example, if you want to try a piece of a rich dessert, share it with the table instead of having one all to yourself.

Lastly, when you're dining out, it can be helpful to plan ahead. Many restaurants have their menus online, allowing you to decide what you will order before you even arrive. This prevents making impulsive decisions based on hunger or the influence of what others are ordering. If you know the restaurant doesn't offer many healthy options, consider eating a small, healthy snack before you go. This way, you won't be overly hungry and can make more controlled food choices.

Making smart choices while dining out is about more than just selecting the right foods. It's about making decisions that contribute to a long-term healthy lifestyle. Remember, managing your cardiovascular health isn't just about the occasional meal but about making consistently beneficial choices. By applying these strategies, you can enjoy your meals out without guilt and with great benefits to your heart health.

Staying Hydrated and Limiting Alcohol Consumption

When we talk about maintaining heart health, two elements that often get overlooked are hydration and alcohol consumption. Both play significant roles in how well our cardiovascular system operates. It's important to understand why staying hydrated is necessary and how alcohol can affect our heart health.

Hydration is crucial for overall health but it specifically supports the cardiovascular system by helping maintain the volume of blood circulating through the body. This makes it easier for the heart to pump the blood. When your body has the right amount of water, your heart does not have to work as hard. Water also helps in transporting nutrients and oxygen to cells, aiding in proper muscle function, and improving the removal of waste products from the body.

What does it mean to stay properly hydrated? It involves consuming an adequate amount of fluids daily. For adults, a general recommendation is about 8 glasses of water a day, but this requirement can vary based on your body size, the climate you live in, your activity levels, and your overall health. Drinking water regularly throughout the day is key. This can be from plain water, fruits, and vegetables that contain high amounts of water, or other beverages. However, it's best to stick with water as it provides hydration without added calories or sugars.

On the other hand, alcohol consumption needs careful management, especially as it pertains to heart health. While moderate alcohol consumption has been noted in some studies to offer certain heart benefits like increasing good cholesterol (HDL), excessive drinking can have adverse effects. It can lead to high blood pressure, irregular heartbeats, and in extreme cases, heart failure.

Limiting alcohol intake is therefore essential. If you choose to drink, doing so in moderation is key. This is typically defined as up to one drink a day for women and up to two drinks a day for men. Yet, even with moderate drinking, it's important to know your own body's response and consult with a healthcare provider, especially if you have existing health issues or take medication that alcohol might affect.

Here are some actionable tips to help you manage hydration and alcohol consumption:

1. Start your day by drinking a glass of water. This simple habit can kickstart your hydration early, setting a good tone for the day.

2. Carry a water bottle with you throughout the day. Having water on hand makes it more likely that you will drink consistently, rather than all at once.

3. Choose water over sugary drinks. This will not only help with hydration but also avoid calorie overload which is beneficial for weight management, a key component in maintaining heart health.

4. Monitor your urine color. If it’s pale yellow, you’re probably hydrated. Darker urine can be a sign of dehydration and a cue to increase

your fluid intake.

5. Set limits for alcohol consumption before social events. Decide how many drinks you'll have ahead of time and stick to your decision to avoid excessive intake.

6. Alternate between alcoholic and non-alcoholic drinks during social gatherings to keep alcohol consumption in check and maintain hydration.

7. Opt for water-rich foods like cucumbers, tomatoes, oranges, and watermelon. These foods can contribute to your daily water intake while providing valuable nutrients.

By being mindful of both hydration and your alcohol consumption, you are taking proactive steps to support your cardiovascular health. This approach not only aids in maintaining a healthy heart but also enhances your overall well-being. Remember, every small step you take can lead to significant health benefits down the road.

Chapter Recap

As we wrap up this chapter on Nutrition for Cardiovascular Health, it's important to revisit the fundamental principles that contribute to a heart-healthy diet and lifestyle. Throughout this chapter, we've explored various aspects of eating and drinking that directly impact heart health. Let's summarize these key points and delve into practical, actionable steps you can take to integrate these principles into your daily life, enhancing both your heart health and overall well-being.

First and foremost, the role of diet in maintaining heart health cannot be overstated. A balanced diet rich in nutrients supports heart function and reduces the risk of cardiovascular diseases. The foods you choose to eat regularly can influence blood pressure, cholesterol levels, and inflammation, all of which are linked to heart health.

Embracing a heart-healthy eating pattern is crucial. This involves focusing on whole, minimally processed foods. Whole grains, lean proteins, healthy fats, and an abundance of fruits and vegetables should form the cornerstone of your diet. These foods provide the necessary nutrients that your heart needs to function optimally.

It's also vital to manage portion sizes and overall calorie intake. Eating too much of even the healthiest foods can lead to weight gain, which is a risk factor for heart disease. Learning to control portion sizes helps in maintaining a healthy weight and improving heart health. Techniques such as using smaller plates or bowls, checking food labels for serving sizes, and listening to your body's hunger cues are effective ways to manage portions.

When dining out, making smart choices can help you stick to a heart-healthy diet. Opt for dishes that are grilled, baked, or steamed rather than fried. Request dressings and sauces on the side to control the amount you consume. These small modifications can make a significant difference in managing your heart health while still enjoying a meal out.

Staying hydrated is essential, and limiting alcohol consumption plays a critical role in cardiovascular health. Water supports the overall function of your body, including your heart. It helps transport nutrients and oxygen to cells, aids digestion, and prevents dehydration. Meanwhile, controlling alcohol intake can help reduce the risk of developing heart disease.

Now, let's turn these concepts into concrete action steps you can start implementing today:

- **Plan your meals:** Each week, take some time to plan your meals. This helps in making informed choices about what to eat and ensures that you have the necessary ingredients to prepare heart-healthy meals.
- **Shop smart:** When grocery shopping, focus on purchasing fresh produce, lean proteins, and whole grains. Avoid the aisles with processed foods and snacks high in sugar, salt, and unhealthy fats.
- **Prepare meals at home:** Cooking at home allows you to control the ingredients and cooking methods. Use heart-healthy oils like olive or canola oil and increase the use of herbs and spices to flavor your food instead of relying on excessive salt.
- **Monitor portion sizes:** Use measuring cups or a kitchen scale to familiarize yourself with recommended serving sizes. This practice can help you avoid overeating, which is crucial for maintaining a healthy weight.
- **Stay hydrated:** Aim to drink at least eight glasses of water a day, more if you are physically active or live in a hot climate. Keeping

a water bottle handy is a practical way to ensure you meet your daily water intake.

- **Limited alcohol intake:** If you choose to drink, do so in moderation. For men, this means up to two drinks per day, and for women, up to one drink per day.
- **Educate yourself:** Continuously educate yourself about cardiovascular health and nutrition. Knowledge is a powerful tool in making lifestyle changes that last.

Implementing these steps can lead to significant improvements in your cardiovascular health. Each small change contributes to a stronger heart and a healthier life. As you make these adjustments, monitor how you feel. You'll likely notice that you have more energy, better digestion, and improved overall health. These positive changes can help motivate you to continue on your journey to a heart-healthy lifestyle.

Remember, the journey to better heart health is a gradual process. It involves making consistent choices that benefit your heart and overall health. By incorporating these practical steps into your daily routine, you are laying the foundation for a healthier, more vibrant life.

In conclusion, embracing a heart-healthy diet is not just about avoiding illness. It's about creating a life full of vitality and longevity. With the right knowledge and actions, you can significantly influence your heart health and enjoy the benefits for years to come.

Understanding the Impact of Stress on Cardiovascular Health

Stress is a condition that affects us all, and its impact on cardiovascular health is significant, especially as we advance in age. When we talk about stress, we refer to the body's response to any demand or challenge that disrupts our normal balance. This response can have various effects on our heart and blood vessels, which are essential components of the cardiovascular system. Understanding these effects is crucial for anyone looking to maintain their heart health and enhance their quality of life.

The heart is a powerful muscle responsible for pumping blood throughout the body. To perform this vital function, the heart needs to be in good condition. Chronic stress can interfere with this by causing several physiological changes that may harm the heart. When stressed, the body releases adrenaline and cortisol, hormones that prepare the body to react to the perceived threat or stressor. This is often referred to as the 'fight or flight' response.

One immediate effect of these hormones is an increase in heart rate and blood pressure. This response is meant to prepare the body to act quickly, but when the stress is constant, having a continually elevated heart rate and blood pressure can lead to serious health issues. High blood pressure, or hypertension, is a significant risk factor for developing heart diseases such as heart attacks or strokes.

Furthermore, stress influences how blood clots, which is a natural process necessary for healing wounds. However, under stress, the body's ability to regulate blood clotting can become skewed, potentially leading to an increased risk of blockages in the arteries. These blockages can cause heart attacks and strokes. Understanding this link is crucial because it highlights why managing stress is so important for heart health.

Chronic stress also affects our behavior, which in turn impacts our cardiovascular health. When people feel stressed, they might turn to unhealthy coping mechanisms such as smoking, overeating, or consuming too much alcohol. Each of these behaviors can increase the risk of developing cardiovascular disease. Smoking, for example, damages the lining of the arteries and contributes to the buildup of artery-clogging plaque. Overeating can lead to obesity and diabetes, which are known risk factors for heart disease. Excessive alcohol intake can raise blood pressure and trigger irregular heartbeats.

Recognizing these links between stress, behavior, and cardiovascular health is a fundamental step in preventing heart diseases. By acknowledging the impact of stress, individuals can take proactive steps towards modifying their stress responses and choosing healthier coping mechanisms. This shift is crucial for anyone looking to protect their heart and improve their overall health as they age.

In conclusion, understanding the impact of stress on cardiovascular health involves recognizing both the physiological changes caused by chronic stress and the behavioral consequences that can further harm the heart. Managing stress effectively not only helps in maintaining a healthy heart but also enhances one's overall well-being and quality of life. This knowledge empowers individuals to make informed decisions about their health and to take actionable steps towards mitigating the effects of stress on their heart.

It is evident that stress management is not just about feeling better in the moment but also about making long-term improvements in heart health. As we continue to explore further stress management techniques in the subsequent sections, remember that each step towards reducing stress is a step towards a healthier heart and a longer, more fulfilling life.

Practicing Mindfulness and Relaxation Techniques

Mindfulness and relaxation techniques are essential tools that help manage stress and enhance overall cardiovascular health. Let's discuss how incorporating meditation, deep breathing, and progressive muscle relaxation not only contributes to stress reduction but also benefits heart health. Understanding these methods and learning how to apply them can make a significant difference in your life, especially if you are looking to manage or prevent cardiovascular diseases.

Meditation is a practice where you focus your mind on a particular object, thought, or activity to train attention and awareness, and achieve a mentally clear and emotionally calm and stable state. For adults over 40, incorporating meditation into daily life can be particularly beneficial. It helps lower stress levels, which in turn reduces the strain on your heart. Meditation can be as simple as sitting quietly for a few minutes each day and focusing on your breath or a mantra. The key is consistency; practicing meditation regularly can help manage stress levels and reduce the risk of cardiovascular disease.

Deep breathing is another technique that plays a crucial role in stress management. It involves focusing on slow, deep, and consistent breaths to help calm the mind and reduce tension. When you breathe deeply, it sends a message to your brain to calm down and relax. The brain then forwards this message to your body. Such breathing exercises can be done at any time of the day and are particularly helpful during moments of heightened stress. This not only helps in managing immediate stress but also has long-term benefits for heart health by reducing blood pressure and promoting better circulation.

Progressive muscle relaxation is a method that involves tensing and then relaxing each muscle group in the body. This technique helps in identifying areas where you hold stress and teaches you how to relax those muscles consciously. Start from the toes and work your way up to the top of your head. By tensing your muscles before relaxing them, you cause a profound sense of relaxation in the muscle, which can help relieve stress and reduce the physical discomfort associated with stress, such as headaches or backaches.

Cultivating present-moment awareness, or mindfulness, is about maintaining a moment-by-moment awareness of our thoughts, feelings, bodily sensations, and surrounding environment. This technique helps in reducing stress by allowing you to realize that stressors are not as immediate as they appear, giving you space and choice in how to respond. Mindfulness can be practiced through simple activities like mindful walking, eating, or even listening. Practicing mindfulness helps in reducing the fight-or-flight response which is often detrimental to heart health.

To integrate these practices into your daily routine, start small. Dedicate a few minutes each morning to meditation. You might sit in a quiet space and focus on your breathing or use a guided meditation app. Incorporate deep breathing exercises during times when you feel your stress levels rising. Take a few deep breaths before entering a stressful situation or when you find yourself caught up in a stressful thought. For progressive muscle relaxation, it might be beneficial to set aside a specific time in the evening as it can also aid in improving sleep quality.

The beauty of these techniques lies in their simplicity and the profound impact they can have on health. By regularly practicing these relaxation methods, not only can you manage your stress better, but you also take an active step towards improving your cardiovascular health. Over time, these practices can lead to significant changes, including lower blood pressure, reduced heart rate, and an overall sense of well-being, which are crucial for anyone looking to manage or prevent cardiovascular diseases.

Remember, the goal is not to eliminate stress entirely but to manage it in a way that doesn't harm your health. Regularly engaging in mindfulness and relaxation techniques provides you with the tools to cope with stress more effectively. By taking control of your stress, you are taking a significant step towards prolonging your life and enhancing the quality of it, especially concerning your cardiovascular health.

In conclusion, mindfulness and relaxation techniques are not just practices but are tools for a healthier life. They require minimal time investment yet offer significant health returns. They are particularly beneficial for adults over 40 who are at a higher risk of cardiovascular diseases. By integrating these practices into your daily life, you can enjoy a more relaxed, healthy, and fulfilling life.

Engaging in Regular Physical Activity for Stress Relief

Physical activity is a powerful tool for managing stress, which, in turn, helps maintain your cardiovascular health. When you engage in regular exercise, your body releases chemicals known as endorphins. These are often referred to as the body's natural painkillers because they help to elevate mood and reduce pain. What's crucial to understand here is the direct impact this has on your stress levels and, as a result, on your heart health.

Exercise also helps by mimicking the effects of stress, like the fight or flight response, and helps your body and its systems practice working together through these effects. This can help reduce the harmful effects of stress. Moreover, when you exercise, your body's central and sympathetic nervous systems communicate to help the body respond to stress. This improves your body's overall ability to respond to stress, making physical activity an essential practice for stress management.

Now, let's talk about specific types of exercises that are particularly effective for relieving stress. Gentle, restorative practices such as yoga and tai chi are excellent options. These exercises focus not only on physical movement but also on breathing techniques and mental practices that help reduce tension and anxiety.

Yoga, for instance, combines physical postures, breathing exercises, and meditation to enhance physical flexibility, mental clarity, and stress reduction. The physical aspect of stretching in yoga can relieve tension in stress-prone areas like the neck and lower back. The breathing practices in yoga help in managing the body's response to stress, making it an excellent choice for heart health.

Tai chi, often described as meditation in motion, is another form of exercise that can significantly aid in stress reduction. It involves a series of movements performed in a slow, focused manner accompanied by deep breathing. Tai chi has been found to decrease stress and anxiety, enhance sleep quality, and improve overall wellbeing, which are vital for cardiovascular health.

Engaging in regular physical activity does not mean you need to undertake intense workouts. Even moderate, gentle exercises can provide these stress-relief benefits without putting undue stress on the body. Activities such as walking or cycling can be highly beneficial. They not only help you stay active but also get you outside, which can be a fantastic stress reliever on its own.

The key is consistency and enjoyment. Choose activities you enjoy, as this will help you stick with a regular exercise routine. It is less about the intensity and more about the regularity. The routine of regular physical activity can itself be a stress reliever. It provides a break from the daily grind, helps regulate your sleep patterns, and can improve your self-esteem.

Incorporating physical activity into your daily life for stress relief doesn’t have to be overwhelming. Start small; perhaps a daily walk or a few yoga poses in the morning. Gradually, as you build your endurance and strength, you can increase the duration and intensity of your activities. It’s important to listen to your body and not overdo it, as pushing too hard can lead to injury, which can be stressful.

To make it more manageable, consider setting achievable goals related to physical activity. Whether it's reaching a certain number of steps each day, attending a set number of yoga classes per week, or simply ensuring you stand up and stretch every hour while at work, setting clear, manageable goals can help you stay on track and make regular physical activity a part of your routine.

As you engage in physical activities, monitor your progress.

Notice if you feel less stressed or have more energy. Keeping track of these changes can motivate you to maintain an active lifestyle. Remember, the goal is to use physical activity as a tool to manage stress, which is a critical aspect of maintaining heart health.

In conclusion, regular physical activity is a crucial strategy for managing stress, which is essential for cardiovascular health. By engaging in exercises like yoga and tai chi, or even simpler activities such as walking, you not only reduce stress but also enhance your overall health and wellbeing. Start slowly, enjoy the process, and gradually integrate these practices into your life to reap their full benefits for your heart and mind.

Nurturing Supportive Relationships and Social Connections

Nurturing supportive relationships and social connections plays a pivotal role in effectively managing stress, which, in turn, benefits cardiovascular health. Why is this support so crucial? Having strong relationships helps reduce the feelings of loneliness and anxiety, which are often associated with increased stress levels. Stress, especially when chronic, can lead to serious heart-related issues, including high blood pressure and irregular heart rhythms.

Let's explore the importance of social support in managing stress. Relationships with family, friends, and the community provide a buffer against the pressures of everyday life. When you share your concerns or thoughts with someone else, it not only relieves the burden you might be carrying alone but also provides different perspectives that might help you see solutions or aspects that you hadn't considered before. This process is beneficial for your emotional well-being and, by extension, your heart health.

What exactly does cultivating meaningful connections mean? It involves actively engaging in relationships where both parties feel valued and supported. It's not enough to just surround yourself with people. The key is to foster relationships that provide mutual benefits through emotional connection, understanding, and respect. These connections can significantly reduce feelings of isolation and stress, contributing positively to your cardiovascular health.

To start building stronger social connections, focus on reaching out to others. It might be as simple as sending a text message or making a phone call to a friend or family member. It's important to make these connections a regular part of your life. Think about joining clubs, groups, or community gatherings that align with your interests. Participating in social activities not only helps you meet new people but also strengthens your existing relationships by engaging in shared experiences.

Building these connections does require effort and time. However, the rewards are immense, not only for your emotional and mental health but also for your physical health. Engaging in social activities can lead to lower levels of stress hormones like cortisol and adrenaline, which are harmful to the heart when they remain elevated over time.

Another aspect of nurturing relationships is being open to receiving support. Many people find it challenging to accept help when they need it, often due to pride or not wanting to burden others. It's important to allow others to offer support. This can make your relationships stronger and provide a sense of community and belonging, which is incredibly beneficial for mental health and stress reduction.

Lastly, remember that nurturing supportive relationships isn't just about taking. It's also about giving. Being there for others can provide a sense of purpose and fulfillment that enhances your own well-being while helping someone else. Supporting others in times of need can strengthen your bonds and create a supportive network that everyone benefits from during stressful times.

In conclusion, prioritizing and nurturing supportive relationships and social connections can significantly reduce stress and improve your cardiovascular health. By taking steps to be both a supportive presence in the lives of others and open to receiving support yourself, you cultivate a network that not only enriches your life but also protects your health. Engage actively with your community, cherish family bonds, and maintain friendships that bring joy and support into your daily life. This approach not only fosters a thriving social life but also constructs a solid foundation for your cardiovascular health.

Creating a Balanced and Fulfilling Lifestyle

Creating a lifestyle that is both balanced and fulfilling is particularly important for anyone, but especially so for adults over 40 who are focusing on managing or preventing cardiovascular diseases. The heart, like any other part of the body, responds to how we live day-to-day. Therefore, it's essential to not only look at diet and exercise but also at the overall approach to living. A balanced lifestyle encompasses various aspects of life, from work and family to recreation and self-care. Let’s break down these elements.

Firstly, prioritizing self-care is not just a trend; it's a necessity for maintaining heart health. Self-care refers to any activity that we do deliberately in order to take care of our mental, emotional, and physical health. Good self-care is key to improved mood and reduced anxiety. It’s not just about treating yourself; it’s making sure that you’re getting enough sleep, that you are eating meals that are nutritious, and that you are exercising regularly. These habits directly impact cardiovascular health by reducing risks like high blood pressure and obesity.

Engaging in enjoyable hobbies and activities is another facet of leading a balanced lifestyle. Hobbies can reduce stress by keeping you engaged in something you enjoy. They provide a break from routine, which can reduce heart rate and improve your overall mood. Whether it's gardening, reading, or painting, hobbies offer a meaningful escape from everyday stress. This isn't just about passing the time; it's about enriching your life and, by extension, enhancing your health.

Another crucial aspect is establishing healthy boundaries. Learning to say no is vital. It isn't about being unhelpful; rather, it's about recognizing what you can realistically handle without feeling overwhelmed. Stress management is critical in cardiovascular health, and overcommitting can lead to stress, anxiety, and ultimately, physical health problems. Setting clear boundaries with colleagues, friends, and even family can help manage the mental load that often leads to stress.

Now, you might wonder how to practically incorporate these concepts into your everyday life. Let's look at some actionable steps. Start with assessing your current lifestyle. What parts of your day make you feel good? What parts don't? Maybe you realize you're spending too much time at work or in front of the TV. Recognize that each part of your day contributes to your overall health. Next, gradually introduce activities that promote well-being. Perhaps you start a new hobby, like knitting or bird watching. Or maybe you decide to spend more time outdoors. These don't have to be big changes; small, consistent actions add up over time.

Additionally, evaluate your social commitments. Are they making you happy, or are they just obligations? If it's the latter, it might be time to politely decline. This is not selfish. It's necessary for your health. Remember, every commitment you make uses up your time and energy. Make sure they are worth both.

In conclusion, creating a balanced and fulfilling lifestyle isn't just about adding more activities to your day. It's about creating quality in your life that supports your physical, mental, and emotional health. As you begin to implement these changes, monitor how they affect your stress levels and overall happiness. Over time, these lifestyle adjustments can lead to significant improvements in cardiovascular health, helping you live a longer, more joyful life.

Finally, the journey to a balanced lifestyle doesn't have to be done alone. Discuss these changes with friends or family who may also want to join you. Support from others can make a big difference in maintaining these healthy lifestyle changes. Remember, the goal is to enjoy life while taking care of your heart and overall health.

Chapter Recap

Having explored various stress management techniques throughout this chapter, it's clear how crucial managing stress is for maintaining cardiovascular health. Let's take a moment to recap the effective strategies we've discussed that can help you prevent or manage heart diseases and improve your overall quality of life.

Firstly, understanding the impact of stress on your heart is foundational. Chronic stress can lead to serious heart problems by increasing heart rate and blood pressure, and by triggering unhealthy coping mechanisms like smoking or overeating. By acknowledging this, you can begin to see why adopting stress reduction techniques is not just beneficial, but essential.

Practicing mindfulness and relaxation techniques such as meditation, deep breathing, and progressive muscle relaxation are not only effective in calming your mind but also have direct benefits on your cardiovascular system. These practices reduce stress hormones in the body, which helps to lower blood pressure and improve heart rate variability, thus enhancing heart health.

Engaging in regular physical activity is another key strategy. Exercise not only helps in reducing stress but also strengthens your heart muscle, improves blood circulation, and helps in maintaining a healthy weight. Activities like yoga and tai chi are especially beneficial as they combine physical movement with mindfulness, enhancing both your physical and mental health.

Maintaining supportive relationships and having a social network can also provide emotional support, which alleviates stress. Whether it's family, friends, or community groups, being connected to others provides a sense of belonging and self-worth, which are important for mental health and resilience.

Lastly, creating a balanced and fulfilling lifestyle is integral. This includes engaging in hobbies, setting healthy boundaries, and learning to say no, which helps in managing stress levels and contributes to a healthier heart.

Now, let’s translate these insights into specific, actionable steps you can begin implementing today to reduce stress and enhance your heart health:

- **Start a Daily Meditation Practice:** Dedicate at least 10 minutes each day to meditation. Begin by finding a quiet space, sitting comfortably, and focusing on your breath. This practice can help in reducing stress and calming your mind.
- **Incorporate Deep Breathing Exercises:** Several times throughout your day, especially during moments of high stress, take a pause to perform deep breathing exercises. Inhale slowly through your nose, hold your breath for a few seconds, then exhale slowly through your mouth.
- **Schedule Regular Exercise:** Aim for at least 150 minutes of moderate aerobic activity or 75 minutes of vigorous activity each week, as recommended by health guidelines. Choose activities you enjoy to ensure consistency.
- **Connect with Others:** Make it a point to regularly spend time with family and friends. Social interactions can help reduce stress levels and provide emotional support.
- **Engage in Hobbies:** Set aside time each week to engage in activities that bring you joy and relaxation, whether it's reading, gardening, or any other hobby that you love.
- **Practice Saying No:** Learn to set boundaries and say no to requests that would overload your schedule or cause undue stress. Remember, it’s okay to prioritize your health and wellbeing.

Implementing these steps doesn't require drastic changes to your lifestyle, but they do require a commitment to consistent practice. Start with small, manageable goals and gradually build upon them as you become more comfortable with these practices. Remember, the journey to improved heart health through stress management is a marathon, not a sprint. Take it one step at a time and be kind to yourself throughout the process.

As we conclude this chapter, reflect on the techniques that resonate most with you and consider how you can integrate them into your daily routine. Managing stress effectively not only improves your cardiovascular health but also enhances your overall wellbeing, paving the way for a healthier, happier life.

Understanding Key Cardiovascular Health Indicators

When it comes to heart health, it's crucial to know and understand certain health indicators that can tell you much about your cardiovascular condition. These indicators include blood pressure, cholesterol, and heart rate. Each of these plays a significant role in your overall cardiovascular health and understanding them can help you manage your heart health effectively.

Blood pressure is a well-known health metric that measures the force of blood pushing against the walls of your arteries. This pressure is crucial because if it's too high, it can make the heart work too hard and contribute to artery damage. It's expressed in two numbers: systolic (the pressure when the heart beats) and diastolic (the pressure when the heart rests between beats). Normal blood pressure is usually considered around 120/80 mmHg. Managing blood pressure is vital because high blood pressure, or hypertension, can lead to severe heart complications such as stroke and heart attack.

Cholesterol is another essential marker for cardiovascular health. It is a fatty substance found in the cells of your body. While your body needs cholesterol to continue building healthy cells, having high cholesterol can increase your risk of heart disease. Your body has two types of cholesterol: LDL (low-density lipoprotein) which is sometimes called 'bad' cholesterol because a high LDL level leads to a buildup of cholesterol in your arteries, and HDL (high-density lipoprotein), known as 'good' cholesterol because it helps remove other forms of cholesterol from your bloodstream. It's important to maintain a proper balance between these two types to keep your heart healthy.

Heart rate, or pulse, is the number of times your heart beats per minute and is a simple measure of how hard your heart is working. In adults, a normal resting heart rate ranges from 60 to 100 beats per minute. Factors like stress, hormones, medications, and how physically active you are can affect your heart rate. An unusually high or low heart rate may indicate an underlying problem and could lead to complications if left unchecked.

The significance of these metrics lies in their ability to provide insights about your cardiovascular health. Regular monitoring of these values allows for early detection of potential health issues, which can be crucial in preventing more severe diseases. For instance, identifying and managing high blood pressure can help prevent a heart attack or stroke, which might otherwise have been fatal. Similarly, by controlling your cholesterol levels, you can reduce the buildup of plaques in your arteries, lowering the risk of heart disease.

Furthermore, understanding these indicators helps you make informed decisions about lifestyle changes. For instance, if you know your cholesterol level is high, you might choose to adjust your diet to include healthier fats and more fiber, which can help lower your cholesterol. Knowing your heart rate can also help you tailor your exercise programs to improve your cardiovascular fitness without overstraining your heart.

Therefore, each of these health metrics offers valuable insights into your heart's health and overall wellness. By keeping track of these numbers and understanding what they mean, you can take proactive steps towards maintaining or improving your cardiovascular health, ultimately leading to a longer, healthier life. This knowledge empowers you to communicate more effectively with healthcare providers and take an active role in managing your health.

It is also worth noting that while these indicators are helpful, they are just part of a bigger picture. Comprehensive health monitoring often includes other factors such as diet, exercise, and genetic history. However, understanding these basic yet crucial indicators is an excellent first step toward heart health awareness and management, setting the foundation for a more in-depth approach as needed.

In conclusion, the importance of understanding your blood pressure, cholesterol, and heart rate cannot be overstated. They are key indicators that can tell much about your heart health and what you can do to manage it. Keeping an eye on these can help you catch potential problems early and adjust your lifestyle to maintain or improve your cardiovascular health. Remember, knowledge is power, especially when it comes to health and wellbeing.

By now, you should feel more informed about these essential

cardiovascular health metrics. Keep these insights in mind, and make sure to discuss any concerns or anomalies you notice with your healthcare provider. Together, you can work towards maintaining a healthy heart and a fulfilling life.

Tracking Progress with Regular Check-Ups and Tests

Keeping track of your cardiovascular health is vital, especially as you age. Regular check-ups and tests are fundamental actions that you can take to ensure you're doing everything possible to prevent or manage cardiovascular diseases. These routine visits to healthcare providers are not only about disease detection; they are also about maintaining a dialogue with your healthcare team, understanding your body better, and making informed decisions about your health.

Scheduling regular visits with your healthcare provider is crucial. It ensures that any potential health issues can be caught early when they are often easier and less costly to treat. During these visits, your doctor will check basic yet essential health indicators such as blood pressure, cholesterol levels, and heart rate. These metrics are critical gauges of your heart's health and overall well-being.

But why are these visits so important? First, they provide a benchmark for you. Knowing your numbers helps you understand where you stand health-wise and what you need to focus on. It's easier to track progress when you have clear, concrete figures to refer to. Also, these visits offer the opportunity for your healthcare provider to review and adjust any treatments or medications you might be taking, ensuring they are still appropriate for your current health status.

Recommended screenings and tests vary based on several factors, including age, family history, and existing health conditions. For instance, if you're over 40, it's generally advised to have your cholesterol checked at least every five years. If you have risk factors for heart disease, more frequent monitoring might be necessary. These tests can provide vital data that helps in crafting a targeted approach to your healthcare.

Risk factors play a significant role in determining the frequency and type of screenings you need. Factors such as smoking, diabetes, obesity, and a family history of heart disease may prompt your doctor to recommend more frequent cardiovascular evaluations. These screenings might include electrocardiograms (ECGs or EKGs), which record the electrical signals in your heart to find irregularities, or stress tests that monitor your heart while you're active.

Another critical aspect of these regular check-ups is that they can motivate you. Seeing improvement in your metrics or stabilizing your condition can be encouraging and reinforce the lifestyle changes you've been making. Conversely, discovering areas where your condition may have worsened can serve as a wake-up call, pushing you to take your health more seriously.

It's not just about the tests themselves, but also about building a relationship with your healthcare provider. These regular interactions create a rapport and a comfort level, making it easier for you to discuss symptoms or concerns that might be troubling you. A good relationship with your healthcare provider boosts your confidence in the care you receive and helps ensure that you're both working towards the same health goals.

Your healthcare provider can also use the information from your tests and your health history to make predictions about potential health risks. This predictive aspect can be crucial for preventive measures. For instance, if your tests show that you're at an increased risk for stroke, proactive steps can be taken to address this, such as adjusting your diet, increasing your exercise, or starting new medications.

In conclusion, maintaining regular check-ups and undergoing recommended screenings are more than just routine parts of healthcare; they are proactive, essential strategies that empower you to take control of your cardiovascular health. These tests provide the data needed to make informed decisions and tailor your health strategies effectively. So remember, staying engaged with your healthcare provider, keeping up with your appointments, and adhering to recommended screenings are all integral parts of managing your cardiovascular health and enhancing your quality of life.

With this comprehensive understanding, you are now better equipped to take active steps towards managing your cardiovascular health. Remember, it's not only about adding years to your life but also life to your years. By regularly monitoring your health through these check-ups and tests, you're taking significant strides in maintaining a healthy heart and a fulfilling life.

Utilizing At-Home Monitoring Devices

Keeping track of your heart health is crucial, especially if you are above 40 or are concerned about cardiovascular diseases. One of the best ways to do this is by using at-home monitoring devices. These devices help you check your blood pressure, heart rate, and other important health metrics without always having to go to a doctor's office.

Let's talk about what these devices are and how they can help you. At-home monitoring devices include things like blood pressure monitors and heart rate monitors. These devices are usually compact, easy to use, and relatively affordable. They provide a way for you to keep an eye on your health daily, which is particularly important if you have a history of heart health issues.

Why are these readings important? Well, keeping track of your blood pressure and heart rate helps you see patterns. These patterns could tell you if your current diet, exercise, and medications are working. Or they might alert you to a potential problem that needs closer examination by a healthcare professional.

First, let's discuss blood pressure monitors. A typical at-home blood pressure monitor wraps around your upper arm and inflates to measure the pressure in your arteries. It's essential to follow the instructions that come with your device to get accurate readings. This usually involves sitting quietly and ensuring the cuff is placed correctly on your arm. Taking your blood pressure at the same time each day can also provide more consistent results.

Now, about heart rate monitors. These can be standalone devices or features included in fitness trackers. They work by sensing your pulse through your skin. For accuracy, it’s important to ensure the device is in direct contact with your skin and that it's neither too loose nor too tight.

Using these devices at home is quite straightforward. Once you have either a blood pressure monitor or a heart rate monitor, or both, you should take readings regularly. Record these readings. You can use a simple notebook or a digital app if you prefer. The key is consistency and accuracy to track your health over time effectively.

Proper technique is crucial for accurate measurements. When measuring your blood pressure, make sure you are relaxed and seated comfortably with your back supported and legs uncrossed. Place your arm on a flat surface so that the cuff is level with your heart. Avoid exercise, caffeine, and smoking at least 30 minutes before taking your measurement.

For heart rate, while most modern devices provide quick readings, it’s still a good idea to sit still during measurements. If you exercise, wait a few minutes after stopping so that your heart rate returns to its resting rate for a stable measure.

It's also worthwhile to learn what the numbers mean. A normal blood pressure reading is usually around 120/80 mmHg, but what's normal can vary slightly from person to person. Similarly, a typical resting heart rate for adults ranges from 60 to 100 beats per minute. Knowing your usual readings can help you spot any unusual changes more quickly.

Lastly, while these devices are incredibly helpful, they are not substitutes for professional medical advice. They are best used as tools for regular monitoring that can help you stay informed about your heart health. It's always good practice to discuss your findings with your healthcare provider, especially if you notice significant changes in your readings.

By taking these steps, you are taking control of your health. Regular monitoring can provide peace of mind and is a good way to detect potential health issues early. This proactive approach to health monitoring is particularly beneficial as we age, helping us maintain better overall health and a higher quality of life.

Keeping a Health Journal and Documenting Changes

Recording daily metrics such as blood pressure, heart rate, and other factors is a vital habit for anyone focused on managing or preventing cardiovascular diseases. A health journal serves as a personal record of your health journey. It helps you and your healthcare provider notice patterns and make adjustments to your lifestyle or treatment plan. When you write down details like what you eat, how much you exercise, and how you feel, it can reveal valuable insights into what impacts your heart health.

Starting a health journal might seem simple, but it is essential to understand how to do it effectively to benefit your cardiovascular health. The first step is to choose a medium that you are comfortable with. This could be a traditional notebook, a digital app, or even a spreadsheet on your computer. The key is consistency, so pick a format that you will stick to every day.

Each day, record your blood pressure and heart rate. These are critical metrics for understanding your cardiovascular health. Blood pressure readings give you insights into the pressure in your arteries and heart, while heart rate provides data on how hard your heart is working. If you are using medication to manage these metrics, note down the time and dosage as well.

In addition to these measurements, track your physical activity. Write down the type of exercise, duration, and how intense the activity felt. This information can be very helpful, especially when you discuss your exercise routine with your doctor. They might adjust your activities based on how they affect your heart rate and overall health.

Diet is another crucial aspect to monitor in your health journal. Document everything you eat and drink, noting the time and portions. This record will help you and your healthcare provider understand the relationship between your diet and your heart health. Over time, you may notice that certain foods impact your energy levels, blood pressure, and general wellness.

Symptoms should also be recorded in your health journal. This includes any chest pain, fatigue, dizziness, or unusual shortness of breath. These entries can be critical for your doctor to diagnose potential issues early. Writing down your feelings and symptoms daily provides a comprehensive view of your health and how it changes over time.

Try to reflect on your mood and any stressors in your daily entries. Emotional health is closely linked to cardiovascular health. Stress can affect blood pressure and heart health, so noting your emotional state can be as important as recording physical health metrics.

Lastly, review your health journal regularly with your healthcare provider. This review can happen during regular check-ups, or more frequently if you're managing a specific health issue. Your doctor can help you interpret the patterns in your journal, suggest changes, and provide tailored advice. This collaborative approach can significantly enhance the effectiveness of your health monitoring.

By keeping a detailed health journal, you are taking an active role in managing your cardiovascular health. This practice helps you recognize what improves or harms your well-being, allowing you and your healthcare provider to make informed decisions. It can lead to better management of symptoms and a healthier lifestyle overall. Regularly updating and reviewing your health journal can transform it into a powerful tool in your journey towards heart health.

Collaborating with Healthcare Providers

When it comes to maintaining your cardiovascular health, one of the most effective strategies is working closely with healthcare providers. This partnership is critical because it allows for tailored advice and adjustments to your health plan based on your specific needs and medical history.

Firstly, it's essential to establish a relationship with a primary care physician or a cardiologist who understands your health background and the goals you're aiming to achieve. This medical professional acts as your main point of contact for managing your cardiovascular health. They play a crucial role in interpreting the health data you collect, whether it's from at-home monitoring devices, lab tests, or physical examinations.

During each visit with your healthcare provider, it's advisable to come prepared. This means having a list of questions or concerns about your cardiovascular health, as well as any symptoms you might be experiencing. It's also helpful to bring a record of your blood pressure readings, cholesterol levels, and any other relevant health metrics you've been tracking. This information provides a comprehensive view of your health and helps your doctor make informed decisions.

Your discussions should focus on understanding the results of your tests and check-ups. If your blood pressure has changed since the last visit, or if your cholesterol levels aren't where they should be, your doctor can explain what these changes mean. More importantly, they can help you understand what can be done to improve these metrics.

Developing a personalized health plan is another crucial aspect of your collaboration with your healthcare provider. This plan should outline specific steps you can take to manage or improve your cardiovascular health. It might include dietary recommendations, exercise, medication changes, or other lifestyle adjustments. Your provider can set realistic goals and timelines, making the plan actionable and tailored to your individual health status.

Regular follow-ups are vital. These allow you and your doctor to assess whether the health plan is working or if it needs adjustments. Consistent communication with your healthcare provider not only helps in tracking your progress but also in maintaining motivation. It’s reassuring to know that a professional is overseeing your journey and can provide support when needed.

When health issues arise, timely intervention can make a significant difference. If you experience new symptoms or if your self-monitored data show unusual results, contact your healthcare provider immediately. Quick responses can prevent complications and adjust your health plan promptly to address these changes.

Lastly, always ensure that any medical advice or plans are clear and understood. If there’s something you don’t understand about your health plan or the reasons behind certain recommendations, ask for clarification. It is crucial that you feel informed and confident about the actions you are taking towards your health. This clarity not only helps in adhering to the plan but also empowers you to make informed decisions about your health care.

In sum, collaborating effectively with healthcare providers is a proactive approach to managing cardiovascular health. It ensures that the measures you are taking are not only effective but also specifically suited to your needs. This partnership enables you to navigate the complexities of health care with confidence, backed by professional guidance and support.

Chapter Recap

Throughout Chapter 8, we've explored various aspects of monitoring health metrics crucial for managing and preventing cardiovascular diseases. Understanding your health indicators and keeping track of them is not just a routine, it's a fundamental part of maintaining your heart health and overall wellness. Let’s reiterate the importance of these activities and provide you with a clear, actionable checklist to ensure you stay on top of your cardiovascular health.

Blood pressure, cholesterol levels, and heart rate are more than just numbers; they are insights into your body’s condition. Regular monitoring of these metrics can give you early warnings of potential health issues or provide reassurance that your lifestyle choices are paying off. Whether through visits to your health care provider or using at-home monitoring devices, keeping an eye on these figures is essential.

Consistency is key when it comes to health monitoring. Regular check-ups allow professionals to catch issues before they become severe. Home monitoring devices have made it easier to stay informed about your health without constant trips to the doctor. Yet, understanding how to use these devices correctly is crucial to ensure the data you gather is accurate.

Recording your daily health metrics can provide you with a treasure trove of actionable data over time. This helps not only in self-assessment but also provides your healthcare provider with detailed information, enabling a more tailored approach to your health care plan. A health journal serves as a valuable tool in this regard, helping track progress and understand the impact of lifestyle changes on your health.

Now, let's turn these insights into action. Below is a checklist designed to help you maintain and improve your cardiovascular health through effective monitoring:

- **Schedule Regular Check-Ups:** Make appointments with your healthcare provider at intervals recommended based on your age and health condition. These regular interactions ensure any changes in your health are noted promptly.
- **Invest in a Home Monitoring Device:** Consider purchasing a reliable blood pressure monitor and perhaps a wearable device to track your heart rate and activity levels. Ensure you understand how to use these devices accurately.
- **Maintain a Health Journal:** Start a journal to record your daily

metrics along with any symptoms or unusual feelings. Note down medication intakes, dietary habits, and exercise routines to see correlations between lifestyle and health.

- **Review and Reflect:** Periodically review the data you've collected. Look for trends or changes, and consider discussing these with your healthcare provider to adjust your health management plans as necessary.
- **Stay Informed:** Keep yourself educated about cardiovascular health. Understanding the implications of your metrics will help you make informed decisions about lifestyle changes.
- **Engage with Your Healthcare Provider:** Share your findings and concerns with your doctor. Effective communication with your healthcare provider enhances the care you receive and helps tailor your health strategies more precisely to your needs.

Taking these steps will not only help you keep a vigilant eye on your cardiovascular health but will also empower you to take control of your well-being. Remember, the goal is not just to prevent or manage disease but to enhance the quality of your life, allowing you to enjoy more active, fulfilling years ahead.

As we conclude this chapter, remember that each small step you take is a building block towards a healthier heart. Regular monitoring, combined with informed, proactive health decisions, lays the foundation for longevity and a better quality of life. Keep pushing forward, keep monitoring, and most importantly, keep striving for a healthier you.

Understanding the Connection Between Sleep and Cardiovascular Function

Sleep plays a crucial role in maintaining overall health, and particularly, heart health. During sleep, your body goes through processes that repair and restore organs, including the heart. The heart rate slows, blood pressure drops, and breathing stabilizes, which reduces stress on the heart and allows it to recover from the day's activities. This nightly restoration helps to regulate hormone levels, manage stress responses, and reduce inflammation, all of which are crucial for cardiovascular health.

Good sleep is not just about quantity but also quality. Achieving deep, restorative sleep stages is vital. These stages are when the most significant body recovery occurs. During these deeper stages of sleep, particularly during slow-wave sleep, critical hormones are released. These hormones include growth hormones essential for tissue growth and repair, which also benefit the heart muscles and the vascular system. Therefore, ensuring a good sleep pattern is not merely a part of a healthy lifestyle but a fundamental element in heart disease prevention strategies.

Sleep deprivation can lead to a number of cardiovascular risk factors becoming more pronounced. When the body misses out on sleep, it experiences physiological stress, leading to increased blood pressure and heart rate, both of which put extra strain on the heart. Chronic sleep deprivation has been linked to a variety of serious health issues, including hypertension, coronary heart disease, and even myocardial infarction (heart attack).

When you do not sleep enough, your body produces higher levels of stress hormones such as cortisol. High cortisol levels can lead to increased glucose production, which not only contributes to weight gain but also increases the risk of type 2 diabetes, a significant risk factor for cardiovascular diseases. Furthermore, poor sleep has been associated with higher levels of inflammation, another risk factor for heart disease and other health issues. Inflammation can lead to the development of atherosclerosis, where arteries become clogged with fatty deposits, which can eventually lead to heart attacks and strokes.

In summary, sleep is not a luxury but a necessity, especially when considering cardiovascular health. Ensuring you get adequate, quality sleep each night is a powerful way to reduce the risk of heart disease. It helps to manage weight, lower stress hormone levels, reduce inflammation, and maintain normal blood pressure and heart rate. Paying attention to sleep hygiene and addressing sleep disorders early can significantly contribute to a heart-healthy lifestyle.

By understanding the connection between sleep and cardiovascular function, you can take proactive steps to improve your sleep. This not only enhances your overall health and well-being but directly contributes to reducing your risk of cardiovascular disease. Prioritizing sleep is a simple yet effective way to care for your heart.

As part of a comprehensive approach to heart health, managing sleep patterns emerges as a fundamental aspect. Now, knowing the critical role sleep plays and the adverse impacts of sleep deprivation, you can better appreciate why a good night's rest is more than just resting the mind, it's about nurturing the heart. Taking control of your sleep is a significant step towards achieving and maintaining optimal cardiovascular health, thereby improving your quality of life and longevity.

Establishing a Consistent Sleep Schedule

Setting a consistent sleep schedule is crucial for maintaining good heart health. When we talk about a consistent sleep schedule, we mean going to bed and waking up at the same time every day. This regularity helps your body's internal clock, also known as the circadian rhythm, to stabilize. A stable circadian rhythm improves sleep quality, which in turn, can reduce the risk of cardiovascular diseases.

Why is this stability so important? Our bodies thrive on routine. By waking up and going to bed at the same times, even on weekends, you help your body anticipate and prepare for sleep. As adults over 40, maintaining a schedule helps counteract the natural changes in sleep patterns that may occur with aging, such as earlier bedtimes and wake times or waking up throughout the night.

To start setting your sleep schedule, choose a bedtime that allows you to get at least 7-8 hours of sleep each night. Consider what time you need to wake up, based on your daily responsibilities, and work backward from there. If you need to wake up at 6 AM, for example, plan to go to bed around 10 PM or 11 PM. Once you've chosen your times, stick to them as closely as possible every day.

Creating a relaxing bedtime routine is also part of establishing a consistent sleep schedule. A routine signals to your body that it's time to wind down and prepare for sleep. This routine can include activities like reading a book, taking a warm bath, or listening to soothing music. It's best to avoid screens from televisions, smartphones, and computers, as the blue light emitted can interfere with your ability to fall asleep.

Begin your routine about 30 to 60 minutes before your set bedtime. This gives you ample time to relax your mind and body. Avoid heavy meals and caffeine close to bedtime as they can disrupt your sleep. Instead, opt for a light snack if you are hungry. Foods like bananas, a small cup of yogurt, or a piece of whole-grain toast can be perfect as they are not too heavy but will prevent hunger pangs at night.

Consistency is key, not just in timing but in your nightly activities. Try to perform the same relaxing activities in the same order each night. This consistency reinforces the signal to your body that it's time to sleep, making it easier to fall asleep quickly.

Stick to your schedule diligently. It might take some time for your body to adapt, especially if your previous sleep schedule was irregular. However, after a few weeks, most people find that they start feeling sleepy at their scheduled bedtime and wake up naturally at the right time in the morning.

Remember, the goal of a consistent sleep schedule is not just to improve sleep but also to enhance overall heart health. Good sleep doesn't just make you feel better. It lowers stress, regulates mood, and decreases the risk of serious health issues, including heart disease. Therefore, by committing to a regular sleep-wake cycle, you're taking a significant step toward better health and longevity.

In conclusion, setting a consistent sleep schedule is a proactive strategy to enhance your quality of life by improving sleep quality and reducing the risk of cardiovascular diseases. Follow these steps meticulously, and you are likely to see beneficial changes in both your sleep patterns and heart health. This simple, yet effective approach can provide a foundation for a healthier lifestyle as you age.

Creating a Sleep-Conducive Environment

When it comes to enhancing your heart health through better sleep, the environment in which you sleep plays a crucial role. Think about the bedroom where you sleep each night. This space, ideally, should be a sanctuary that promotes relaxation and deep, restful sleep. Here we will discuss how to optimize this environment by adjusting the temperature, lighting, noise levels, and investing in a comfortable, supportive mattress and pillows.

First, let's talk about the temperature in your bedroom. It's important to keep the room at a comfortable temperature to facilitate good sleep. Generally, experts recommend setting your bedroom temperature around 65 degrees Fahrenheit (18 degrees Celsius). This might seem slightly cool, but it helps your body's core temperature decrease, which is a signal for your body to start preparing for sleep. If the room is too hot or too cold, it may interfere with this natural process, making it harder for you to fall asleep and stay asleep.

Lighting is another critical factor. Excessive light exposure, especially blue light from screens like smartphones, tablets, and televisions, can disrupt your body's ability to prepare for sleep because it inhibits the production of melatonin, a hormone that helps regulate sleep. To create a sleep-conducive environment, minimize light in your bedroom. Use heavy curtains or shades to block light from outside, and try to limit the use of electronic devices in the hour before bed. Perhaps consider using lamps with softer light and, if necessary, a sleep mask to block out any residual light.

Noise levels also significantly impact the quality of your sleep. Noise can prevent you from falling asleep initially, and sounds during the night can wake you from sleep. You can manage noise by using earplugs or a white noise machine. A white noise machine produces a consistent, soothing sound that can help mask disruptive noises such as traffic or a partner's snoring.

Now, let's consider the comfort of your bed. A high-quality mattress and pillows that provide adequate support are worth the investment. The right mattress will support your body in a neutral position, where your spine has proper alignment and you are not forced into uncomfortable angles. Remember, we spend about one-third of our life sleeping, so it's crucial to ensure your bed helps rather than hinders the quality of your sleep. If you often wake up with pains or aches, it might be time to consider a new mattress.

Similarly, the right pillow can make a significant difference in your sleep quality. The pillow should support the natural curve of your neck when you are lying down. There are various types of pillows available including memory foam, feather, or cervical pillows designed specifically to support the neck. Take the time to find one that feels comfortable and supports your sleeping position, whether you sleep on your back, side, or stomach.

By making these changes, you create an environment that is more conducive to sleep. Remember, good quality sleep is not just about quantity. It's also about the quality of your sleep environment. As you improve your sleep environment, you might find that you not only sleep longer but also feel more rested and rejuvenated the next day. This has a direct and positive impact on your cardiovascular health, contributing to overall wellbeing and longevity.

Investing time and effort into creating the right sleep

environment can dramatically improve your sleep quality, which in turn, benefits your heart health. It's one of the most straightforward actions you can take with a substantial return on investment for your health. Consider this as part of your broader strategy to manage or prevent cardiovascular diseases. Every night of good sleep is a step towards a healthier heart.

Addressing Common Sleep Disorders

Sleep is crucial for heart health. Many adults face sleep challenges that can impact their cardiovascular system. Today, we will talk about common sleep disorders such as sleep apnea, insomnia, and restless leg syndrome. Understanding these conditions is the first step toward better sleep and heart health.

Let's start with sleep apnea. Sleep apnea is when your breathing stops and starts while you sleep. This can happen many times during the night. It's not just about snoring or feeling tired, it's a serious issue. Sleep apnea makes your heart work harder, which can lead to high blood pressure and other heart problems. If you snore loudly, wake up often during the night gasping for air, or feel very tired during the day, you might have sleep apnea.

It's important to see a doctor if you think you have sleep apnea. They can tell you to do a sleep study. This study can be done in a sleep clinic or at home. The results will help your doctor understand your sleep patterns and breathing. Treatment might include using a CPAP machine at night. This machine helps keep your airways open while you sleep, which helps you breathe better.

Next, let's discuss insomnia. Insomnia means having trouble falling asleep or staying asleep. This problem can make you feel tired and stressed. Over time, stress and lack of sleep can hurt your heart. With insomnia, you might find yourself lying awake, worrying and watching the clock. You might wake up too early and not be able to go back to sleep. If this happens a lot, it's called insomnia.

There are ways to help manage insomnia. Try going to bed at the same time each night. Make sure your bedroom is quiet and dark. Avoid caffeine and heavy meals before bedtime. If stress is keeping you awake, consider talking to a counselor. They can help you manage your stress. Sometimes, doctors prescribe medicine to help with sleep. However, it's best to try other methods first, like changing your sleep habits.

Lastly, we have restless leg syndrome (RLS). This is when you feel a strong need to move your legs while resting. It often happens in the evening when you are sitting or lying down. Moving your legs provides temporary relief. RLS can make it hard to fall asleep and stay asleep. It's annoying and can lead to tiredness during the day, which is not good for your heart.

Iron deficiency or nerve problems can cause RLS. Your doctor might check your iron levels or look for other health issues. Sometimes, medicines help control the urge to move your legs. Lifestyle changes, like regular exercise and avoiding caffeine, also help.

If you notice signs of these sleep disorders, do not ignore them. Talk to your doctor. Managing these sleep problems can help you sleep better. Better sleep improves your heart health. It also makes you feel more rested and ready for the day.

Remember, the goal is not just to sleep, but to sleep well. Your heart will thank you for it. Start by noticing how you sleep and how you feel during the day. Bring any concerns to your doctor. Together, you can work on a plan to improve your sleep and protect your heart.

To conclude, dealing with sleep disorders is a key part of keeping your heart healthy. Whether it's using a CPAP machine for sleep apnea, setting a regular bedtime for insomnia, or managing RLS symptoms, each step you take can lead to better sleep and a healthier heart. Start taking action today for better sleep tonight and healthier heart tomorrow.

Implementing Relaxation Techniques for Better Sleep

To enhance our sleep quality, especially when concerned about heart health, it's beneficial to incorporate certain relaxation techniques into our nighttime routine. Effective relaxation not only helps in falling asleep quicker but also enhances the depth and quality of sleep. Let's explore some easy-to-implement methods that can be integrated into your evening routine, aimed at setting you up for a restful night, which is crucial for maintaining cardiovascular health.

Firstly, deep breathing exercises are a standout amongst relaxation techniques due to their simplicity and effectiveness. To practice deep breathing, find a comfortable place where you can sit or lie down without interruptions. Close your eyes and slowly inhale through your nose, allowing your chest and lower belly to rise, and then exhale gradually through your mouth. Each breath cycle should ideally last six to eight seconds. Try to focus solely on your breathing. This method helps reduce stress levels, calming both the mind and body, preparing you for sleep.

Another accessible technique is meditation, which involves sitting quietly and paying attention to your breath, a specific word, or phrase. Meditation can reduce bedtime anxiety and create the right mindset for sleep. Start with just five minutes near bedtime and gradually increase the duration. It's about finding a personal rhythm and pattern that soothes your mental state.

Gentle stretching exercises can also profoundly impact sleep quality. Stretching helps release muscle tension and promotes physical relaxation. Some simple stretches include neck rolls, shoulder shrugs, and leg extensions. Each stretch should be held gently for 15 to 30 seconds, allowing muscles to relax progressively. Remember, the goal is to release tension, not to enhance flexibility or engage in intense physical activity right before bed.

Avoiding stimulating activities and electronics before bedtime is also crucial. This includes avoiding work-related emails, exciting or dramatic television programs, and social media browsing at least an hour before bed. The blue light emitted by screens interferes with the production of melatonin, the hormone responsible for regulating sleep cycles. Instead, consider reading a book or listening to calm music, which can significantly help in winding down.

Implementing these relaxation techniques regularly can lead to profound improvements in sleep quality. Improved sleep not only supports heart health but also enhances overall well-being. Make these practices a part of your nightly routine and observe the benefits over time. Remember, consistency is key in reaping the full benefits of any health-related practice. By incorporating these simple yet effective strategies into your life, you are taking a significant step towards improving both your cardiovascular health and your quality of life.

Begin tonight. Choose one or two techniques to start with, and gradually build up your routine. Tailor your approach to what feels most relaxing to you. Whether it's deep breathing, meditation, gentle stretching, or reducing screen time, each step you take is a positive stride towards better health and better sleep.

Chapter Recap

Sleep is crucial for maintaining good heart health. Over the previous sections, we explored various aspects of sleep and its direct influence on cardiovascular function. We discussed how adequate sleep acts as a restorer and guardian of your heart's health. Now, let's consolidate what we've learned into practical, actionable steps that you can start implementing tonight to promote better sleep and, consequently, better heart health.

First, recall the importance of establishing a consistent sleep schedule. Your body thrives on routine. Going to bed and waking up at the same time every day helps regulate your body's internal clock, or circadian rhythm. This rhythm influences your cardiovascular health by managing blood pressure and heart rate. Here's what you can do:

- Set a fixed bedtime and wake-up time that allows for 7 to 9 hours of sleep daily.
- Even on weekends or days off, try to stick to your scheduled sleep times to keep your heart rhythm regular.

Next, creating a sleep-conducive environment is equally vital. The environment in which you sleep can significantly affect the quality of your sleep. Here are some steps to optimize your bedroom:

- Keep your bedroom dark. Use blackout curtains or an eye mask to block out light.
- Maintain a comfortable temperature, ideally between 60-67 degrees Fahrenheit.
- Reduce noise pollution. Consider a white noise machine if you cannot control external noises.
- Invest in a good quality mattress and pillows to support your body and align your spine.

Addressing common sleep disorders is another critical step. Disorders like sleep apnea, insomnia, and restless leg syndrome can severely impact your sleep quality and, by extension, your heart health. Here are specific actions you can take:

- Be aware of the signs of sleep disorders, such as snoring, prolonged insomnia, or daytime fatigue.
- Consult a healthcare provider for a proper diagnosis and treatment plan if you suspect a sleep disorder.

Implementing relaxation techniques before bed can also enhance your sleep quality. These help calm your mind and prepare your body for sleep, reducing the time it takes to fall asleep and improving sleep quality. Try these techniques:

- Practice deep breathing or meditation each night before bed for 10 to 15 minutes.
- Incorporate gentle stretching or yoga poses to relax your muscles.
- Avoid stimulating activities and screens at least an hour before your bedtime.

Finally, let's talk about your pre-sleep routine, which can significantly influence your heart health through better sleep. A relaxing pre-sleep routine helps signal to your body that it is time to wind down and rest. Here's a simple routine you might consider:

- One hour before bed, dim the lights in your home and turn off electronic devices to reduce blue light exposure.

- Have a warm, non-caffeinated drink like herbal tea to increase internal body warmth which can help induce sleep.
- Read a book or listen to calming music to help clear your mind from the day's stresses.

By incorporating these practices into your daily routine, you take proactive steps to enhance your sleep quality. Remember, each small change you make contributes significantly to your overall cardiovascular health and longevity. Start tonight, pick one or two actions from above, and gradually build more healthy sleep habits into your life. Your heart will thank you for it.

Ensuring good sleep isn't just about preventing discomfort; it's a fundamental part of maintaining your heart's health and your overall quality of life as you age. Take these steps seriously and make sleep a priority. It's a major part of caring for your heart and ensuring you have many healthy, active years ahead.

Celebrating Progress and Milestones

When it comes to maintaining your cardiovascular health, setting goals can be a beacon, guiding you through your journey to better heart health. Whether you are trying to prevent heart disease or manage existing conditions, having clear, achievable goals is crucial. Goals act like milestones on the road, giving you direction and something to aim for.

It is beneficial to differentiate between short-term and long-term goals. Short-term goals are like stepping stones that will lead you to your ultimate, long-term aspirations. For example, a short-term goal could be walking 30 minutes a day, five days a week. This is achievable and manageable. On the other hand, a long-term goal might be to reduce your cholesterol levels significantly within a year.

Each goal you set should be specific, measurable, attainable, relevant, and time-bound, often referred to as SMART. Specific goals clearly define what you intend to do; measurable goals allow you to track your progress; attainable goals ensure that the targets are within your reach; relevant goals tie into your larger health objectives; and time-bound goals keep you focused within a specific timeframe.

As you reach these goals, it is vital to acknowledge and celebrate your success. Recognizing your achievements, no matter how small, can significantly boost your motivation. This could be as simple as telling a friend about your progress or rewarding yourself with a healthy treat or new fitness gear. The act of celebrating reinforces your commitment and the positive behavior that led to the achievement.

Rewarding yourself also reinforces the joy associated with achieving these health milestones. When you feel good about what you've accomplished, you're more likely to continue. This positive reinforcement loop can be the key to sustained long-term changes in your lifestyle. It makes the journey enjoyable and something to look forward to.

To keep track of your progress, consider maintaining a health diary or using a digital app. Record your daily activities, food intake, mood, and any significant changes you notice. Periodically reviewing this diary will help you see the progress you've made over time. It serves not only as a motivational tool but also as a way to identify areas that may need more attention or adjustment.

In conclusion, setting achievable goals and celebrating every progress point on the way are essential strategies in managing your cardiovascular health. These practices keep you motivated and committed to your health journey, making the process rewarding and effective. As you continue to meet and set new goals, remember that each step forward is a vital part of your journey toward a healthier heart and a better quality of life.

Identifying and Overcoming Potential Obstacles

As adults over the age of 40 striving to prevent or manage cardiovascular diseases, a crucial aspect is to recognize potential obstacles that might impede progress. Identifying these challenges is the first step toward developing strategies to overcome them. Why is this important? Because foreseeing difficulties allows you to prepare adequately and maintain your journey towards improved longevity and quality of life more effectively.

One common obstacle many face is the lack of immediate results. When changes in diet, exercise, or lifestyle do not show quick outcomes, it can be discouraging. To handle this, setting realistic expectations is essential. Understand that cardiovascular health improvement is a gradual process. It helps to keep track of small improvements; perhaps you can walk a bit longer without feeling tired, or your blood pressure readings improve slightly.

Another challenge that frequently arises is the disruption of routines. Life events such as family gatherings, holidays, or even changes in work schedule can disrupt your exercise and eating habits. Proactively planning can help manage these disruptions. For instance, if you know a busy period is approaching at work, try scheduling shorter, more intensive workouts, or if a holiday is coming up, plan how you will handle your diet and exercise in advance.

Setbacks are also a part of any long-term health journey. It's natural to have days or even weeks where you're not able to stick to your health goals. What's important is how you respond to these setbacks. Instead of viewing them as failures, reframe them as opportunities for growth and learning. Analyzing what led to the setback can provide valuable insights into what adjustments might be necessary in your approach.

For example, if you find you're consistently missing your workout sessions, it might be time to reconsider the type of exercise you are doing. Perhaps the intensity or the timing of the exercise is not fitting well with your current lifestyle. Adjusting these aspects can make your regimen more manageable and enjoyable, increasing the likelihood of sticking to it.

Developing proactive coping strategies is another key element in overcoming obstacles. This involves anticipating potential problems and having a plan to deal with them. If emotional eating is a challenge, strategies such as keeping a food diary or practicing mindfulness can be helpful. It can also be beneficial to have a list of activities, such as walking or a hobby, that you can turn to instead of eating when you feel stressed.

It is also beneficial to have support from friends, family, or even a professional such as a dietitian or a personal trainer. They can offer motivation and advice, and help you stay accountable to your goals. Joining a community, whether online or in person, where members share similar health goals can also provide support and encouragement.

Lastly, continually educate yourself about cardiovascular health. Knowledge is a powerful tool. Understanding the specifics of cardiovascular diseases and how lifestyle factors contribute to them will equip you with the why and how of managing and preventing these conditions. When you know the reasons behind recommended practices, it becomes easier to adopt and stick to them.

To sum up, overcoming obstacles in maintaining cardiovascular health involves a mix of realistic expectation setting, proactive planning, learning from setbacks, developing coping strategies, seeking support, and ongoing education. Each of these elements plays a crucial role in not just facing the challenges head-on but turning them into stepping stones for your health journey. By anticipating these challenges and preparing to deal with them, you enhance your ability to maintain motivation and continue making progress towards a healthier heart and a better quality of life.

Cultivating a Positive Mindset and Self-Compassion

One of the most important steps in managing and preventing cardiovascular diseases as you age is cultivating a positive mindset and practicing self-compassion. This isn't just about feeling good; it's about creating a mental environment where your physical health can thrive. Understanding and applying these principles can significantly influence how you handle the ups and downs of maintaining cardiovascular health.

First, let's explore what it means to have a positive mindset. A positive mindset involves looking at your life and your health in a way that emphasizes the good and minimizes the negative. This doesn't mean ignoring problems or health symptoms. Rather, it's about focusing on your abilities and what you can do to improve or maintain your health. When you keep your mind focused on positive outcomes, you are more likely to engage in behaviors that contribute to those outcomes, such as eating a balanced diet or maintaining a regular exercise regimen.

Practicing self-compassion is equally crucial. Self-compassion means treating yourself with the same kindness and understanding you would offer a good friend in a similar situation. Often, adults over 40 can be hard on themselves, especially after a setback like missing a few days of exercise or indulging in unhealthy eating. Instead of engaging in negative self-talk, which can be demotivating, self-compassion encourages you to acknowledge the slip-up and move forward without judgment.

To start practicing these concepts, focus first on self-acceptance. Accepting yourself does not mean complacency. Instead, it means recognizing your current state without criticism. Acknowledge that everyone has limitations and that progress takes time. When you accept yourself, you set the stage for improvement because you are not wasting energy on feeling inadequate. You can say to yourself, "I am not where I want to be, but I accept where I am now as part of my journey."

Avoiding negative self-talk is another actionable strategy. Negative self-talk often involves telling yourself things you would never say to someone you care about. These might include phrases like "I'm too lazy to get healthy," or "I always fail at diets." To combat this, try to catch yourself in the act of negative self-talk, and replace those thoughts with more constructive ones. For example, instead of saying "I can't stick to a diet," you could say, "I haven't found the right approach yet, but I'm working on understanding what suits me best."

Embracing a growth mindset is another key element. A growth mindset, a term popularized by psychologist Carol Dweck, is the belief that your abilities can be developed through dedication and hard work. This view creates a love of learning and a resilience that is essential for great accomplishment. When it comes to cardiovascular health, a growth mindset helps you see challenges, like learning to cook heart-healthy meals or establishing a new exercise routine, not as insurmountable obstacles, but as opportunities to expand your skills and knowledge.

Viewing challenges as temporary is an extension of the growth mindset. When faced with a setback, remind yourself that this is temporary and that you have the power to overcome it. For instance, if you find it hard to motivate yourself to exercise, remind yourself that you are just in a rut, and you have gotten out of ruts before. This can help reduce the feeling of being overwhelmed and increase your motivation to take action.

Now, let's put these ideas into practice. Begin by setting aside a few minutes each day to reflect on your thoughts and feelings about your health. Identify any patterns of negative self-talk and actively work on reframing these thoughts more positively. You might write down your typical negative thoughts and next to them, write a more compassionate or realistic way to think about the situation.

Additionally, make a commitment to acknowledge every small success along your health journey. Celebrated successes, no matter how small, can include things like choosing a salad over a less healthy option, walking an extra ten minutes, or even managing your stress more effectively than usual. Acknowledging these victories can reinforce your positive mindset and encourage more healthy behaviors.

Lastly, remember that cultivating a positive mindset and practicing self-compassion are ongoing processes. There will be days when it's more challenging than others, and that's okay. The important thing is to keep moving forward, making adjustments as needed, and always striving to treat yourself with kindness and understanding. Over time, these mental practices will become a natural part of your lifestyle, supporting your cardiovascular health and your overall well-being.

Building a Support System and Accountability

When it comes to preventing or managing cardiovascular diseases, it's not just about what you eat or how often you exercise. A crucial component often overlooked is the support system surrounding you.

This is particularly vital for adults over 40, as having a solid network not only motivates you but can significantly affect your resilience and ability to maintain healthy habits over time.

Creating a supportive environment involves surrounding yourself with people who encourage and uplift you. This could be family members, friends, or colleagues who understand your health goals and respect the choices you make to reach those goals. These individuals become your cheerleaders, celebrating small victories with you and helping you stay on track. This sense of community is essential, as it fosters a positive atmosphere that makes your journey less isolating.

Moreover, consider the role of an accountability partner. This is someone who holds you responsible for your commitments. They could be a friend who checks in regularly on your progress, a personal trainer at your gym, or even a healthcare professional like a dietitian or a nurse. The key is to choose someone reliable and honest, who won't hesitate to provide constructive feedback and remind you of your targets when you stray.

Another way to build your support system is by joining a support group. This could be a local community group that meets weekly, or an online group where members share experiences, challenges, and resources. These groups provide a platform for learning from others who might be at different stages of their health journey. For instance, you might find someone who has successfully managed their blood pressure through diet and exercise, and their story could inspire you to follow a similar path. Furthermore, sharing your own struggles and successes makes your journey tangible and helps you see the progress you're making, which can be incredibly motivating.

It is also important to ensure that these interactions and relationships are positive and uplifting. Negative influences, even from well-meaning individuals, can sometimes discourage you from your goals. It's beneficial to have clear discussions with your support group about what kind of support you appreciate and what is not helpful, ensuring that the advice and encouragement you receive aligns with your needs and health goals.

Participating actively in these supportive networks also encourages you to reciprocate the support, fostering a community of mutual care and encouragement. This reciprocity can enhance your commitment to your health goals, as helping others often increases your motivation to stay on course in your own journey.

It's also helpful to set shared goals with your support group or accountability partner. This could involve setting a collective walking goal, preparing healthy meals together, or attending health-related workshops as a group. Shared goals not only make the activities more enjoyable but also reinforce your commitment, as you wouldn't want to let your group down.

In addition, technology can play a supportive role in your health journey. Numerous apps and digital tools are designed to track your progress, remind you of your goals, and even connect you with online communities who share similar aims. Using these tools can add an extra layer of accountability and support, providing you with data-driven insights and access to a wider community of support.

Remember, the road to managing or preventing cardiovascular disease does not have to be walked alone. Building a strong support system and having accountable relationships are pivotal steps towards maintaining your motivation and achieving your health goals. By investing time in fostering these supportive connections, you are setting yourself up for a healthier, more supported journey towards cardiovascular health.

Lastly, always consider reevaluating the dynamics of your support system. As your health journey progresses, your needs might change, and the support you require might evolve as well. Regular check-ins with yourself and your support group can ensure that the support system remains effective and continues to serve your best interests.

By prioritizing and actively building a network of support, you are not just looking after your physical health, but also enhancing your mental and emotional wellbeing. This comprehensive approach to health not only aids in the management of cardiovascular diseases but also improves your overall quality of life, ensuring that you can enjoy your days fully, surrounded by people who care about your wellbeing.

Regularly Reassessing and Adjusting Goals

In the journey towards better cardiovascular health and longevity, it's vital that you regularly reassess and adjust your goals. This practice is not just about staying on track, but also about adapting to the changes in your body, lifestyle, and circumstances that naturally occur as you age.

Why is it so crucial to reassess your goals? Life changes. A goal that was suitable a few months ago might not be fitting today. Maybe you've reached that goal already, or perhaps it has become unattainable or irrelevant due to changes in your health or personal circumstances. It's not just about altering your targets when things don't go as planned but also about recognizing and adjusting to positive changes.

How do you go about this process? First, set a regular schedule for evaluating your goals. This could be every few months or annually. The key is consistency. During these evaluations, look critically at what you've achieved so far and what has changed in your life and health. Are the goals still challenging yet achievable? Are they still relevant?

Next, consider the flexibility of your goals. Life is unpredictable. Your responsibilities at work or home may change, health issues can arise, or new opportunities might present themselves. If your goals are too rigid, they can become sources of frustration instead of motivation. Make sure your goals can bend a little with the winds of change rather than breaking at the first gust.

Adjusting your goals might mean setting new limits for what you can achieve now that you have more experience or knowledge about what works best for your body. It could also mean scaling back if you've been pushing too hard and risking injury. This part of the process is about honest self-assessment and being realistic with what you can achieve, given your current circumstances.

Remember, the main aim is not just to extend your life but to improve the quality of it. This means setting goals that enhance your well-being and happiness. Perhaps initially, your goals were heavily focused on physical health metrics like blood pressure or cholesterol levels. Over time, you might find it beneficial to include goals related to mental health and emotional well-being, such as managing stress or improving sleep quality.

It's also helpful to document your goal-setting and reassessment process. Keeping a journal or log where you can reflect on your progress and the changes you're making can be incredibly beneficial. This record not only serves as a reminder of how far you've come but also helps you understand your patterns of success and areas needing improvement.

Moreover, don't overlook the importance of seeking feedback during your reassessment. This could be from medical professionals, like your doctor or a cardiologist, or from family and friends who understand your health journey. They can provide insights that you might overlook and can help reassess your goals from a fresh perspective.

Finally, always align your goals with actionable steps. It's not enough to simply decide you want to lower your cholesterol. You need to lay out a clear plan of how you're going to achieve this. Will you adjust your diet, increase your physical activity, or possibly seek medication? Detail these steps and set mini-goals that will help you achieve the broader objective. This breakdown not only makes the task seem less daunting but also allows for small victories along the way, keeping you motivated.

In conclusion, the practice of regularly reassessing and adjusting goals is a cornerstone of managing and preventing cardiovascular disease effectively. It ensures that your efforts are aligned with your current health status and life situation, allowing for a personalized approach that is both realistic and flexible. By setting regular reviews, being open to change, and aligning goals with actionable steps, you can maintain motivation and continue making progress towards a healthier heart and a better quality of life.

Chapter Recap

As you have navigated through the various strategies and insights shared in this chapter, it is essential to pull together the key takeaways and translate them into practical steps that you can incorporate into your life. This will ensure that you maintain motivation and resilience on your journey to better cardiovascular health. Let's summarize the strategies and move forward with concrete action steps.

Firstly, acknowledging and celebrating your progress is crucial.

It doesn't matter how small or big your milestones are; each step forward is a victory. This might involve setting a personal record for daily steps, consistently taking your medication, or choosing a salad over a burger during lunch. Recognizing these wins reinforces positive behaviors and bolsters your motivation.

Secondly, anticipate and prepare for potential obstacles. Life is unpredictable, and challenges to your heart health journey are inevitable. Whether it's a busy week with no time for exercise or a family event centered around unhealthy foods, planning for these challenges can help you manage them better when they arise. Developing coping strategies in advance can make all the difference.

Thirdly, cultivating a positive mindset and practicing self-compassion are your allies. Be kind to yourself when things don't go as planned. Understand that setbacks are not failures but opportunities to learn and grow. A positive mindset will help you view these challenges as temporary and surmountable.

Building a strong support system is also vital. Surround yourself with people who encourage and motivate you. This could be family members, friends, or even a community group. People who share your goals can offer practical advice, emotional support, and a gentle push when needed.

Regularly reassessing and adjusting your goals ensures they remain relevant and achievable. This might mean setting new benchmarks as your fitness improves or finding alternative strategies if your current ones are not yielding results. Flexibility in your approach will keep you engaged and responsive to your body's changing needs.

Now, let's make these concepts actionable. Here are steps you can take immediately to apply the insights from this chapter:

- **Set Specific Goals:** Write down three specific, measurable, achievable, relevant, and time-bound (SMART) goals related to your heart health. An example could be, "Walk 10,000 steps a day, five days a week, for the next month."
- **Create a Reward System:** Decide on a way to reward yourself for meeting each goal. Maybe it's a movie night or purchasing a small item you've wanted. Rewards strengthen your commitment to your health goals.
- **Identify Possible Obstacles:** Write down at least three potential challenges you might face in achieving your goals and outline a strategy for overcoming each one. For instance, if bad weather may prevent a walk, plan to use a treadmill or do an indoor exercise video instead.
- **Engage Your Support Network:** Share your goals with at least one person who will hold you accountable. This might be a friend, family member, or a health coach. Check-in with them weekly to report on your progress.
- **Journal Your Journey:** Keep a daily or weekly journal of your progress. Note your feelings, successes, and areas of difficulty. This reflection can provide valuable insights into what

adjustments might be necessary.

- **Review and Reset:** At the end of each month, review your progress towards your goals. Celebrate the successes and understand the shortfalls. Adjust your goals for the next month based on this review.

In conclusion, the journey to improved cardiovascular health is ongoing and dynamic. It requires dedication, adaptability, and a positive outlook. By following these steps, you equip yourself with tools to stay motivated and overcome any setbacks. Remember, each step you take is a part of a larger journey towards a healthier heart and a better quality of life.

Recapping the Key Principles of the Heart Health Journey

Understanding the relationship between intermittent fasting, exercise, and lifestyle is crucial in managing and preventing cardiovascular diseases. Intermittent fasting is not just about skipping meals; it's a structured approach to eating that alternates between periods of eating and fasting. This method helps reduce weight, improves metabolic health, and lowers the risk of heart diseases. By integrating exercise into this regimen, you enhance your body's ability to manage blood sugar and cholesterol levels, further protecting your heart.

Lifestyle factors such as sleep, stress management, and smoking cessation are also part of this interconnected system. Each aspect of your lifestyle either supports or undermines the others. For example, poor sleep can make it harder to stick to your fasting schedule or find motivation for physical activity. Similarly, high stress can lead to unhealthy eating habits and reduced physical activity, which might negate the benefits of intermittent fasting and exercise.

Therefore, adopting a holistic approach means recognizing how these elements are linked. It involves more than just following a diet or exercise routine; it's about creating a balanced system where healthy eating, physical activity, and good lifestyle choices work together to improve your cardiovascular health.

Reinforcing the Importance of a Holistic Approach to Cardiovascular Well-being

A holistic approach to your heart health is essential. This means not just focusing on one aspect, such as diet, but looking at your overall lifestyle. Why is this approach effective? It addresses all the contributing factors to cardiovascular health, which often interact in complex ways. For instance, stress affects your eating habits and exercise routines, while the quality of your diet can influence your stress levels and physical health.

Implementing a holistic approach could include regular physical check-ups, maintaining a balanced diet rich in fruits, vegetables, and lean proteins, regular physical activity, and techniques for stress management such as meditation or yoga. It also means making informed decisions about your health, such as choosing to walk or bike rather than drive, or opting for healthier food choices when dining out.

When you look at heart health through a holistic lens, you’re more likely to sustain positive health behaviors. This is because you're not just focusing on isolated actions but integrating heart-healthy habits into a comprehensive lifestyle that supports overall well-being. This integration makes it easier to stick with healthy behaviors, as they become part of your daily routine rather than exceptions.

Remember, the journey to improved heart health is gradual and requires consistent effort. Small, consistent changes in your diet, exercise, and other lifestyle areas can lead to significant health improvements over time. By focusing on the interconnected nature of lifestyle factors and adopting a holistic approach to health, you can significantly enhance your cardiovascular well-being and overall quality of life.

By reaching the end of this section, you now understand the importance of viewing your heart health as a complex interplay of various factors rather than isolated elements. Embrace this holistic framework and take proactive steps towards a healthier heart and a better life. This understanding not only helps in preventing heart diseases but also plays a significant role in managing existing conditions more effectively. Each small step you take is a building block towards a heart-healthy lifestyle.

Encouraging Readers to Take Action and Embrace Change

Now is the time to prioritize your heart health and embark on making significant changes in your lifestyle that will not only improve your day-to-day life but could also extend it. Throughout this book, we've explored various elements that contribute significantly to cardiovascular health, including the advantages of intermittent fasting and regular physical activity. It is essential to recognize that understanding these concepts is only the first step. The true journey begins when you decide to take action and integrate these practices into your life.

Conclusion

Many adults over the age of 40 face increased risks for cardiovascular diseases due to various factors such as lifestyle choices, past habits, or even genetics. However, it's never too late to make adjustments that can substantially alter the course of your health. By choosing to prioritize your heart health now, you're not just choosing to live longer; you're choosing to live better. Improved cardiovascular health can lead to greater energy levels, better mobility, enhanced mental clarity, and overall a more enjoyable and fulfilling life.

The potential for a better quality of life should serve as a powerful motivator. Think about all the activities you enjoy or the people you love; managing your heart health effectively ensures you can cherish these joys longer and more intensely. It's about making small, manageable changes that collectively lead to significant improvements. This might mean adjusting your diet to include more heart-healthy foods, setting aside time each day for physical activity, or even monitoring your heart health with regular check-ups.

But where should you begin? Start simple. You could begin by reducing the amount of salt and unhealthy fats in your diet. Another actionable step is to incorporate a walk into your daily routine. Gradually increase the pace and distance as you grow more comfortable. If you prefer, join a local gym or a group that focuses on physical activity. The social aspect can also be motivating and enhance your commitment to regular exercise.

Understanding the need to prioritize your heart health is one thing, but taking the necessary steps to make it a reality is another. Commitment is key. Set small, achievable goals and as you meet them, set bigger ones. Each small victory will not only boost your confidence but will also take you one step closer to a healthier heart. Remember, change doesn't happen overnight, and it's okay to have moments of struggle. What's important is that you remain consistent and keep pushing forward.

Moreover, embracing change in your lifestyle for better heart health does not mean you have to do it alone. Engage family members or friends who may also benefit from similar changes. Not only will this provide you with a support network, but it also creates a community of health that fosters collective encouragement and accountability. Additionally, consider consulting with healthcare professionals who can provide personalized guidance based on your specific health needs.

Ultimately, the decision to improve your heart health is yours to make. It is a profound commitment to your future, signaling a desire not only to live longer but to enjoy those additional years fully and actively. By taking action today, you're laying down the foundation for a healthier, brighter future. Let this be the moment you look back on with pride as the beginning of your journey towards a stronger, healthier heart.

You have the tools and knowledge at your disposal, thanks to the insights and strategies shared throughout this book. Now, it’s up to you to put these into practice. Start small, stay consistent, and gradually integrate more substantial changes into your lifestyle. The road to improved cardiovascular health is a journey, but it's one worth taking.

Imagine looking forward to years of life filled with vitality and the ability to engage actively with your loved ones and your passions. By prioritizing and improving your cardiovascular health now, you're taking a significant step towards making this vision a reality. Let's embrace this journey together with optimism and determination.

Providing a Comprehensive Action Plan

Embarking on a journey toward better cardiovascular health involves clear steps. This roadmap is designed to guide you, from the initial assessment of your health to maintaining your achievements. Let's walk through this step-by-step process, ensuring you understand each phase and how it contributes to your overall heart health.

The first step is assessment. This involves evaluating your current cardiovascular health status. You can do this by scheduling a visit with your healthcare provider. During this visit, discuss your family history, any current symptoms you might have, and your lifestyle habits. The goal here is to establish a baseline, which helps in tailoring recommendations that fit your specific needs. Your doctor might suggest some tests such as blood pressure measurement, cholesterol levels, and other heart-related tests. Knowing where you stand is crucial because it sets the direction for your personalized plan.

Once you have a clear understanding of your health status, the next step is to set realistic goals. These should be specific, measurable, achievable, relevant, and time-bound (SMART). For example, if your cholesterol level is high, a goal might be to reduce it to a healthy range within six months by following a specific diet and exercise routine. Goals give you a target to aim for and help motivate you along the way.

After setting your goals, it's time to look at your diet. Nutrition plays a significant role in heart health. Start by gradually introducing heart-healthy foods into your diet. These include fruits, vegetables, whole grains, lean proteins, and healthy fats like those found in nuts and fish. Try to reduce your intake of salt, sugars, and saturated fats, commonly found in processed foods. Plan your meals each week to include these healthier options, making it easier to stick to this new way of eating.

Exercise is another pillar of heart health. If you're not already active, begin with small, manageable steps. You might start with a daily 15-minute walk, gradually increasing the time and intensity as your fitness improves. Aim for at least 150 minutes of moderate aerobic activity or 75 minutes of vigorous activity each week, as recommended by health experts. Regular physical activity helps control weight, reduces the risk of developing other health conditions, and strengthens your heart and cardiovascular system.

Managing stress is also essential in a heart-healthy lifestyle. Chronic stress can lead to high blood pressure, a risk factor for heart disease. Techniques such as deep breathing, meditation, and yoga can be very effective. Schedule regular periods each day to engage in these activities, helping you manage stress more effectively.

Regular monitoring is necessary to track your progress. This could be as simple as noting your daily food intake, keeping a log of your physical activity, or checking your blood pressure at home. These records will help you stay accountable and provide valuable information for your doctor on your next visit. They enable adjustments to be made to your plan, ensuring it remains effective and tailored to your ongoing needs.

Maintaining your new lifestyle is the final step. It's about making these changes a permanent part of your life. This requires persistence and consistency. Continue to educate yourself about cardiovascular health and stay updated with new research. Regular check-ups with your doctor are crucial to ensure you remain on the right track. Also, consider joining support groups or communities where you can share experiences and gain support from others who are on a similar journey.

Success in this journey is not marked by reaching a destination but by continuing to engage in these healthy behaviors day after day. It's about making a lifelong commitment to your heart health. By following this comprehensive action plan, you equip yourself with the knowledge and habits necessary to lead a heart-healthy life. Each step you take builds upon the last, creating a stronger foundation for your cardiovascular health.

This action plan is your roadmap to a healthier heart. Start today by making small changes that will lead to big benefits. Remember, every positive choice adds up, contributing to a healthier and more vibrant life. Embrace this journey with determination and optimism. Your heart is worth it.

Extending an Invitation for Ongoing Support

As we close this journey through understanding and mastering cardiovascular health, it's important to acknowledge that the path to maintaining heart health is ongoing. The commitment doesn't end with the last page of this book. Recognizing the necessity for continued guidance and support, this section is dedicated to directing you towards additional resources that can aid in your journey towards a healthier heart.

First and foremost, seeking out reliable online resources can provide you with up-to-date information and tips related to cardiovascular health. Websites such as the American Heart Association offer a wealth of data, including dietary recommendations, exercise tips, and the latest research findings. These resources are crucial as they provide evidence-based information that you can trust and apply in your daily routine to prevent or manage heart conditions.

Another invaluable resource is support groups. Whether online or in-person, connecting with others who are on a similar health journey can provide emotional support and motivation. These groups offer a platform to share experiences, challenges, and successes. Engaging with a community that understands your struggles and goals can significantly enhance your ability to stick to your health plans and can give you new ideas on how to effectively manage your heart health.

Moreover, considering professional coaching or counseling can be extremely beneficial. A health coach specialized in cardiovascular wellness can offer personalized advice and strategies tailored to your specific needs and health status. They can help you set realistic goals, monitor your progress, and make necessary adjustments to your diet or exercise regimen. This personalized attention can make a significant difference in how effectively you can implement and sustain the changes you need to make.

To facilitate these connections, it is encouraged for you to reach out actively for guidance and support when needed. Taking the initiative to ask questions, seek advice, or simply share your concerns with professionals or peers in support groups can dramatically enhance your understanding and management of heart health. Remember, asking for help is a sign of strength, not weakness, and it plays a crucial role in taking control of your health.

To ensure you continue to receive support, consider subscribing to newsletters from trusted health organizations. These newsletters often contain useful tips, new research updates, and information about community events or webinars that can be beneficial. Keeping informed through these newsletters will help you stay on top of new developments and continue learning ways to improve your heart health long after you have finished reading this book.

Lastly, remember that maintaining heart health is a lifelong commitment. The steps you have learned in this book are just the beginning. Continuing to educate yourself, seeking support, and staying proactive in your health management are key to living a longer, healthier life. With the right tools and a supportive community, you can effectively manage your cardiovascular health and enjoy a better quality of life.

As you move forward, keep in mind that your journey to heart health is unique to you. Tailor the advice you receive to your personal circumstances and always consult with healthcare professionals when making significant changes to your health regimen. With dedication and the right support, you can achieve and maintain optimal heart health.

For more information or to seek additional resources, please visit [www.bhf.org.uk], or contact PROSPECT Cardiovascular Prevention and Rehabilitation (PCPR) Clinic Based in UK and USA on 00447498391793 and 00447482757000 for more personalized support. Your heart health journey continues, and we are here to support you every step of the way.

Remember, the path to better health is not walked alone. Reach out, stay informed, and take control of your heart health with the support of the many resources available to you.

Closing with a Message of Hope and Empowerment

As we draw near the conclusion of our journey through understanding and taking steps towards better cardiovascular health, it's important to recognize the power that comes with knowledge and the willingness to apply it. You, as a reader and an individual seeking to enhance your heart health, have shown remarkable dedication. This commitment to improving your wellbeing is commendable and deserves not just acknowledgment but also encouragement.

The road to better health is often paved with challenges, but the tools and insights shared throughout our discussions provide a robust foundation. These are not just concepts but practical steps that can be integrated into daily life to foster significant improvements in heart health. By embracing these strategies, you harness the capability to not only extend your life but also enhance the quality of your experiences during those years.

Understanding that each step you take towards managing your diet, incorporating exercise, and adjusting your lifestyle contributes significantly to your cardiovascular health is empowering. These changes, while they may require some adjustment, are within your reach. You have the ability to control these aspects of your life, making decisions every day that contribute to a healthier heart.

It's essential to remember that prevention is always more

effective than treatment. By choosing to focus on preventative measures, you reduce the risk of developing heart-related issues later on. This proactive approach is not only beneficial for your physical health but also for your mental wellbeing, as it provides a sense of control and accomplishment.

Let's consider exercise, a key component of heart health. Regular physical activity helps maintain the fitness of your heart just as it would any other muscle in your body. The heart needs to be worked and cared for through activities that keep it active and strong. Whether it's walking, swimming, cycling, or participating in group sports, the type of activity doesn't matter as much as ensuring that you are consistently active.

Similarly, diet plays a critical role in cardiovascular health. Foods rich in omega-3 fatty acids, fiber, and antioxidants contribute positively to heart health, while processed foods and those high in saturated fats do the opposite. Making dietary choices that align with good heart health can seem daunting at first, but once you start, it becomes part of your routine, a part of your life that you can manage and control.

The importance of stress management must also be emphasized. Chronic stress has a deleterious effect on the heart, leading to high blood pressure and other harmful conditions. Techniques such as mindfulness, meditation, and even simple breathing exercises can significantly mitigate these effects. By incorporating these into your daily regimen, you actively reduce the risk factors associated with heart disease.

As we conclude, reflect on the empowerment that comes from being informed and making conscious choices regarding your health. The journey to improved cardiovascular health is ongoing, and while it may require persistence and sometimes tough decisions, it is also filled with hope. Every positive choice is a step towards a longer, more fulfilling life.

Finally, I invite you to carry forward this message of hope and empowerment. Share what you have learned with others who might benefit from it. Your journey could inspire others to begin their own, creating a ripple effect of health and wellness that extends far beyond your immediate circle. This is not just about improving individual lives but also about fostering a healthier, more vibrant society.

Remember, the ability to impact your heart health lies in your hands. Every step you take is a step towards a healthier heart and a more vibrant life. Keep moving forward with optimism, motivation, and the confidence that you are capable of managing your health and transforming your life for the better.

Printed in Great Britain
by Amazon

50127349R00116